COUNTRY
Scents

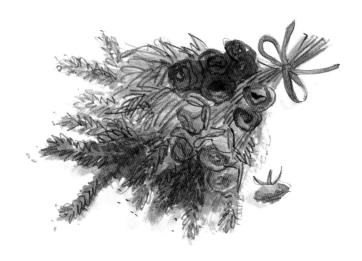

ALAN HAYES

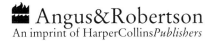

Angus&Robertson
An imprint of HarperCollins*Publishers*

NOTE: Neither the author nor the publisher directly or indirectly dispense medical advice or prescribe the use of the various herbal teas without approval of your health practitioner. The intent is to offer information that you may wish to explore as a natural alternative. Raspberry leaf tea should not be taken during pregnancy without first consulting with your health practitioner, as it may have an abortifacient effect. Allergic reactions from other herbal teas may be found on page 8. Should you use the information on herbal teas, you are prescribing for yourself. This is your right, but the author and publisher assume no responsiblity for your actions.

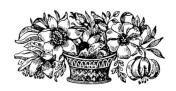

An Angus & Robertson Publication

Angus&Robertson, an imprint of
HarperCollinsPublishers
25 Ryde Road, Pymble, Sydney NSW 2073, Australia
31 View Road, Glenfield, Auckland 10, New Zealand
77-85 Fulham Palace Road, London W6 8JB, United Kingdom
10 East 53rd Street, New York NY 10022, USA

First published in Australia in 1994

Copyright © Alan B. Hayes, 1994

This book is copyright.
Apart from any fair dealing for the purposes of private study, research,
criticism or review, as permitted under the Copyright Act, no part may be reproduced
without written permission. Inquiries should be addressed to the publishers.

National Library of Australia
Cataloguing-in-Publication data:

Hayes, Alan B. (Alan Bruce), 1949-
Country scents.
Updated ed.
ISBN 0 207 18099 7.
1. Herbal cosmetics. 2. Herbs - Therapeutic use. 3. Soap. 4. Herbal teas. I. Title.

646.726

Cover illustration Dianne Bradley
Printed in Hong Kong

5 4 3 2 1
97 96 95 94

Contents

INTRODUCTION

*T*oday there is a growing trend once again towards a more natural lifestyle and the use of natural products. People have begun to realise the importance of living in harmony with nature. The natural benefit of herbs has reawakened the desire to use products that are not harmful to ourselves or planet Earth.

This book shows you how to make your own herbal products. Contained within its pages are down-to-earth recipes for moisturising creams, skin lotions, body oils, shampoos and much more. It takes you step-by-step through each recipe, and shows the ease and simplicity of making the products in your own home. It also deals specifically with maintaining a holistic approach to natural health and beauty.

There are tips for pampering your body, recipes for specific skin problems such as acne, and a list of those herbs most beneficial for relaxing baths and taking care of your hair. This book also gives you methods of extracting your own herbal essences, how to dry herbs for future use, plus a guide to creating your own fragrant herb garden and a dictionary of beneficial plants.

And to maintain that healthy bloom, remember that it is equally important to eat well and exercise regularly. A good diet of natural foods, such as herbs, fresh fruit and vegetables, is essential. Some herbs in particular have certain beneficial effects on the organs and systems of the body. For this reason I have devoted a chapter to these herbs and how they contribute to a healthier lifestyle.

This is not just a recipe book, but a key to a healthier, more natural way of life.

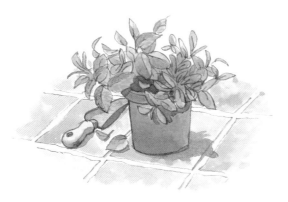

General Advice

❖

About the Recipes

Throughout this book I have endeavoured to keep the various preparations as pure and simple as possible. As a result of this you won't end up with a cream or lotion that looks like a commercial product. In most instances the various preparations will tend to be plain, with no real colour at all. To add colour is to sacrifice purity for superficial appearance.

Occasionally a number of the recipes (in particular, facial creams), include the addition of a 'fragrant oil'. While this does improve the smell of some of the creams and lotions, it is not absolutely necessary as the recipe is equally acceptable unperfumed.

Ingredients

If an ingredient or term is unfamiliar to you it can be looked up in the Glossary at the end of the book. Each listing is simply and clearly explained.

Always use distilled water in all recipes, including the preparation of herb or flower waters. This is essential to prevent creams and lotions turning rancid, since tap water contains chemicals and impurities which might interfere with the action of the herbs and other ingredients.

Many of the recipes' ingredients include extracted or pure essential oils, herbal infusions, flower waters, decoctions and herbal and floral vinegars. Instructions for making them are given in Chapter Eight.

Most recipes call only for small amounts of a particular infusion, flower water or decoction to be used, so more than likely you will have a quantity left over. Never waste it: leftovers can be added to your evening bath and will exert their beneficial effects on your body skin.

A Word of Advice

When making the various recipes you will need only basic kitchen equipment, plus other odds and ends that are usually found there. However, before you start, there are a number of precautions that should be taken, so as not to contaminate or mar the various preparations:

➤ do not use aluminium, metal, or non-stick pans for boiling or steeping herbs and flowers, or for the preparation of herbal recipes, as they may chemically react with the natural ingredients. Use only stainless

steel or enamel pans for boiling and ceramic or glass pots for steeping;
- all equipment must be kept spotlessly clean, and preferably used only for the preparation of herbal recipes. This safeguards the products from contamination by foodstuffs and other foreign substances. Again, do not use metal or aluminium, and always use a wooden spoon to stir, particularly when heating up ingredients;
- sterilise all containers and their lids. Preferably use glass jars to keep the cosmetics in, as they are easier to sterilise.

Glass jars and metal lids should be thoroughly washed and rinsed clean, then placed in a saucepan of water, brought to the boil, and allowed to simmer for ten minutes. Remove from heat and leave containers in hot water until ready for use.

Plastic containers and lids should be thoroughly scrubbed, rinsed clean with warm water, then filled with hot water and the lid replaced. Stand for ten minutes, then invert the container and stand for a further ten minutes;

- adequately label everything you make — don't rely on memory;
- an electric beater can be used to homogenise the ingredients instead of beating with a spoon;
- warm herbal water and oils before adding to melted wax when making creams;
- always use fresh herbs unless dried herbs are specified. If using dried herbs, choose only those with good aroma and colour.

Keeping Herb and Flower Waters

It is important to keep all herbal waters as fresh as possible. Being organic, and with no preservatives, they will deteriorate — some more quickly than others, depending on the plants used. However, there are exceptions such as lavender, which has good keeping qualities due to its antiseptic properties. Other infusions will keep quite well in a cupboard if blended with an odourless alcohol such as vodka or gin, or if a few drops of benzoin tincture (friar's balsam) are added.

If you add 5–10 ml (⅓ fl oz) of alcohol to every 300–500 ml (16 fl oz) of infusion, or 3–4 drops benzoin tincture to every 300 ml, this will extend the keeping qualities of the mixture. However, should you wish to make larger quantities and ensure that the infusion will last indefinitely, add one part alcohol to two parts infusion, stand for 12 hours, then drip through filter paper.

Unpreserved infusions and shampoo preparations will keep from seven days to seven months in the refrigerator, providing their containers have been sterilised and are spotlessly clean. But don't leave them and forget about them — check regularly to make sure they haven't gone rancid.

Keeping Lotions and Creams

Lotions and creams made with lemon juice will keep for several weeks in a cool, dark cupboard. Add 8–12 drops of lemon juice to any of the lotions or cream recipes, unless already included. The addition of 3–4 drops of benzoin tincture will also extend their keeping qualities.

It must be remembered, however, that, unlike commercially manufactured cosmetics, these preparations are not intended to be long lasting. The quantities specified in the various recipes ensure that there is only sufficient cream or lotion for your immediate needs.

Recipes

To simplify the recipes the following abbreviations have been used:

g   grams
ml   millilitres

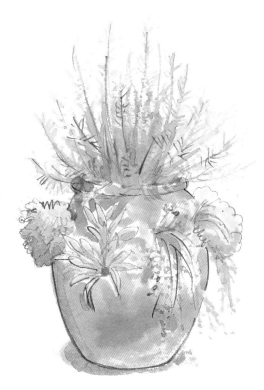

Allergic Reaction to Herbs

Because of the increase in skin sensitivities and allergic reactions, and the fact that no cosmetic can claim to be totally hypoallergenic, it is important to be mindful of any new substance or ingredient before use. Lotions and creams can be patch tested on the underside of the forearm, and if a reaction occurs — reddening, blistering, burning or itching of the skin — the offending ingredient can be substituted with another herb that has the same beneficial effect.

If your skin does react and you have discovered through a process of elimination that this is due to the inclusion of lanolin or glycerine, substitute completely with beeswax. This will in no way affect the beneficial properties of the preparation.

Some vegetable and essential oils can irritate sensitive skins, particularly on the face and around the neck. Those which might cause allergic reactions are:

almond oil	bay leaf oil
bergamot	pennyroyal
peppermint	rosemary (hypersensitive people only)
geranium (all types)	spearmint
parsley (large doses)	sage
neroli	lavender (very large doses)
thyme	

Herbs which might cause allergic reactions are:

cowslips	ivy
lime (linden) blossoms	lovage
nettles	pennyroyal
violet leaves	

Other ingredients which could cause a reaction are:

cocoa butter	cucumber
glycerine	lanolin

Herbs which might cause allergic reactions when taken as a tea are:

angelica — may produce sugar in the urine in people with a tendency to diabetes

juniper — overuse of the berries can cause irritation and inflammation of the kidneys

rosemary — should not be taken as a tea during pregnancy as it may affect the circulation

sage — excessive use as a tea may cause inflammation of the mucous membrane of the mouth in hypersensitive individuals

CHAPTER ONE
The Face of Nature

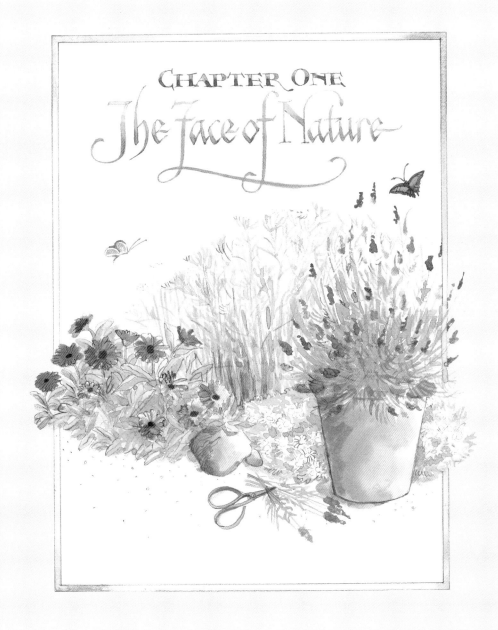

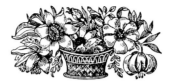

*Y*our face is one of the most expressive parts of your body, the mirror of your personality, so it is very important to keep it in top condition.

Before you start you must learn to observe your skin's requirements, which will alter according to your state of health, your diet, and the climate in which you work and live. Once you have become familiar with your skin you can then work out a routine to suit your skin type and its individual needs.

The three basic steps in facial skin care are cleansing, toning and moisturising. With each of these steps there are simple procedures that should be adhered to:

- Be gentle when applying preparations; don't irritate or drag on the skin.
- Smooth lotions on, then blot off any excess after about fifteen minutes.
- Avoid extreme heat or cold; both are bad for skin.
- Clean facial skin regularly.
- Don't overcleanse or clog the pores with huge lashings of moisturising cream.
- Avoid harsh toning.

Before preparing your natural skin care products, it is important to be aware of your skin type and the best way to look after it. The four main skin types are: dry, oily, sensitive and normal. Most people do not fall into a single category but are a combination of dry and oily, with oily areas being found along the hairline, forehead, and a central strip down the face. If there is a large difference between skin types, you must first determine the problem areas and then treat them separately — first using a moisturiser formulated for the appropriate areas.

Normal skin is clear, supple and soft; neither too dry nor too oily, and is not overly sensitive to sun, climate or environment.

Dry skin looks dull, feels tight after washing and needs constant protection to avoid flaking and peeling.

Sensitive, delicate skin reacts badly to sunlight or irritants by burning. It does not tan well and will quite easily develop rashes, blotches or spots when exposed to new substances.

Oily skin will often feel soft and supple, but look shiny and is usually prone to outbreaks of spots.

Cleansing the Face

❖

A daily cleansing routine is the first and single most important step to skin care. It entails removal of all the grime and dirt which accumulates on your skin every day. If you are living in the city, or work there, this accumulation of grime and dirt is far more severe than if you enjoy country air.

Natural cleansers are usually a combination of beeswax, oil, water and various beneficial herbs which melt when massaged on to your skin. This massage action frees particles of dirt, grime, grease and stale make-up. After use the cleanser must be wiped off with a soft piece of cloth so that it doesn't become absorbed into your skin along with the suspended particles of grime.

To complement your daily cleansing program it is essential that you thoroughly cleanse your face once a week either by using a steam bath, face mask or face scrub. Do not use any of these methods more frequently unless you have persistent blemishes, as they dry the skin.

Facial Steam Bath

There would be very few people who haven't used an inhalation at some time or another to help clear a stuffy nose or a head cold. A facial steam bath is taken the same way and promotes perspiration, which encourages the pores to expel impurities and dirt. This leaves your face feeling clean and refreshed.

Choose from any of the following herbs appropriate to your needs:

Cleansing and Soothing	chamomile, nettle, rosemary, thyme and yarrow
Tightening Facial Pores	sage, peppermint, elder flower and yarrow
Skin Healers	comfrey and fennel
Ingrained Dirt, Spots and Acne	thyme, fennel, chamomile, nettle and dandelion

To prepare your steam bath place 2 teaspoons of dried herb, or 20 drops of herbal oil, in a ceramic bowl and add 1 litre (32 fl oz) of boiling water. Hold your face over the bowl and cover your head with a towel large enough to form a tent and prevent the steam from escaping. Steam cleanse for no longer than 10 minutes, ensuring that you do not overexpose your skin to the heat.

Facial steams should not be used at all on very dry skin because it is usually too sensitive to heat. The steam and heat may also affect people with overly sensitive skin or dilated red veins, and those who have heart trouble, experience difficulties in breathing or suffer from asthma. If you have any of these problems, use a face mask instead. Face masks will not only cleanse and soothe facial skin, but will help to draw out hard-to-remove grime from clogged pores, as well as blackheads and dead skin.

CHAMOMILE CLEANSER AND TONIC

This mask is suitable for all skin types
and will leave your face
feeling fresh and clean.

4 cups chamomile
1 teaspoon fennel seeds
1 tsp fennel leaves

Place the herb mixture in a pan and cover with boiling water. Simmer for about 10 minutes, or until the herbs combine into a thick mash, then set aside to cool. Spread mask, while still warm, over a piece of sterile cotton or lint and apply to your face, avoiding eyes and mouth. Leave for 15 minutes, then wash off with lukewarm water, rinsing well. Splash the skin with cold water and pat dry with a soft towel.

HONEY WHEATGERM CLEANSER

A nourishing cleansing mask
that is especially good for
removing blackheads.

5 tablespoons honey
1 tablespoon wheatgerm oil

Mix both ingredients together and spread on face. Leave on for 15 minutes, then wash off with lukewarm water, rinsing well. Splash the skin with cold water or apply a herbal toner to close the pores.

GRAPE FACE PACK

❖

A cleansing and revitalising mask ideal for dry skin.

100 g (3½ oz) seedless green grapes
5 ml (⅙ fl oz) clear honey
1 egg yolk

Wash the grapes, rub them through a fine sieve and mix with the rest of the
ingredients. Spread over the face and neck and leave on for 15 minutes.
Rinse off with lukewarm water and apply a herbal toner.

OILY SKIN TREATMENT

❖

1 ripe pear
2 tablespoons powdered milk
4 tablespoons finely ground yarrow
linseed oil
cider vinegar

Mash the pear and mix with the rest of the ingredients, but only use
sufficient oil and cider vinegar to make a thick paste. Leave on for 15
minutes, then rinse off with lukewarm water. Splash the skin with cold water
and pat dry with a soft towel.

This mask will purify, stimulate and revitalise tired-looking skin, giving a
healthy glow to your complexion.
TIP: To treat oily skin apply a little lemon juice with cotton wool before
washing the face, taking care to avoid contact with the eyes.

DANDELION TOILET WATER

❖

*Wash the face night and morning with this, when not using
facial steams or face packs, to remove grime and keep the skin
healthy and supple.*

generous handful of dandelion leaves
1 litre (32 fl oz) boiling water

Add dandelion leaves to water in an enamel or stainless steel pan and boil for
half an hour. Remove from heat, cool, then strain through muslin cloth.
Store in a tightly-sealed bottle in the refrigerator for up to 7 days.

Face Scrubs

These cleanse in exactly the same way as a face mask, the only difference being that they can easily be applied whilst taking a shower, and need only a few minutes to massage into the skin. Perfect for people in a hurry.

O ATMEAL F ACE S CRUB

4 tablespoons fuller's earth
2 tablespoons oatmeal
4 tablespoons mixture of finely ground herbs —
chamomile, fennel seed, mint and rosemary
12 drops lemon juice
aloe vera juice
wheatgerm oil
natural yoghurt
1½ tablespoons brewer's yeast

Mix together all ingredients, adding sufficient yoghurt, oil and aloe vera juice to form a thick paste. Apply to your face and neck, avoiding the area around the eyes and any broken skin. Massage lightly into your skin for 5 or 6 minutes and then remove by rinsing thoroughly.
Tone and moisturise after your shower.

Cleansing Creams and Lotions

A VOCADO C REAM C LEANSER

10 g (⅓ oz) anhydrous lanolin
5 g beeswax
65 ml (2 fl oz) avocado oil
10 ml (⅓ fl oz) wheatgerm oil
40 ml (1½ fl oz) chamomile infusion (see Chapter Eight)
3 drops tincture of benzoin

Melt the lanolin and wax in a double pan over low heat. When completely liquid stir in the oils and infusion until well blended. Remove from heat, pour into a ceramic bowl, add tincture of benzoin and stir vigorously until cool and of a creamy texture. Store in a sterilised, screw-top glass jar.

Apply a small amount to facial skin morning and night, massaging in gently, and then remove all traces with a soft piece of clean cloth.

YOGHURT AND HONEY LOTION
❖

A gentle cleansing milk that exerts natural antiseptic and bleaching properties, ideal for oily skins.

15 ml (½ fl oz) natural yoghurt
2 teaspoons clear honey
1 teaspoon pure lemon juice

Mix all the ingredients together and massage gently into facial skin, using small circular motions. Then remove all traces with a soft piece of clean cloth. Rinse face two or three times with cold water and pat dry with a soft towel.

LAVENDER CLEANSING LOTION
❖

Use this lotion to cleanse both normal and disturbed skin.

50 ml (1½ fl oz) jojoba oil
30 ml (1 fl oz) almond oil
20 ml (⅔ fl oz) wheatgerm oil
10 drops essential oil of lavender (see Chapter Eight)

Thoroughly mix the four oils together and store in a tightly-sealed amber-coloured glass bottle in a cool, dark cupboard. Always shake well before use.

Pour a little of the oil into the palm of one hand and warm by rubbing the palms together. Smooth over the entire face and neck and then lightly massage into the skin with small, circular movements.

Gently wipe away all traces of the cleansing lotion with a flannel wrung out in hand-hot water, rinsing at least twice more in hot water. When all traces of oil have been removed splash the skin with cold water and pat dry with a soft towel.

Cream as a Skin Cleanser

Cream makes an excellent skin cleanser. Smooth well into your skin, leave for a few minutes, and then rinse with tepid water and then with cold. Pat your face dry with a towel.

If your skin tends to be oily, add a few drops of lemon juice to the cream.

Toning the Face

❖

Toning the facial skin is the next important step in your daily skin care routine. Because cleansing opens the pores slightly, it is important to use an astringent to close them again. At the same time it will remove the last traces of grease, dead cells and grime, and firm the skin.

Skin tonics also redress the skin's pH balance and so normalise the skin's mantle, and those formulated for oily skin remove excess sebum and also restrict sebum secretion.

TONER FOR TIRED, SAGGING SKIN
❖

1 tablespoon chamomile
1 tablespoon comfrey or elder flower
2 tablespoons rosemary
2 tablespoons nettle
500 ml (16 fl oz) white wine vinegar

Put the herbs into a large, wide-mouthed jar that has an airtight stopper. Gently warm the wine vinegar and pour over the herbs. Seal the jar and leave in a sunny location for about 2 weeks. Shake the contents every day and then test at the end of 14 days by placing a little vinegar on the back of your hand. If it doesn't smell herby enough, repeat the procedure with a fresh batch of herbs.

Strain through muslin cloth and then dilute 20 ml (⅔ fl oz) of vinegar to every 150 ml (5 fl oz) of distilled water. This type of toner will last indefinitely. Store in a glass bottle with a tight-fitting lid.

OILY SKIN*
❖

2 teaspoons dried sage
2 teaspoons dried yarrow
1 teaspoon dried rosemary
1 teaspoon dried, chopped lemon grass

* Replace wine vinegar with cider vinegar

SENSITIVE SKIN

1 teaspoon dried fennel seed
3 teaspoons dried rose petals
2 teaspoons dried elder flower

DRY SKIN

2 teaspoons dried rose petals
2 teaspoons dried nettle
1 teaspoon dried elder flower
1 teaspoon dried, chopped lemon grass

SPOTS AND ACNE

2 teaspoons dried thyme
2 teaspoons dried lavender
2 teaspoons dried, chopped lemon grass

Prepare and use as for toner for *Tired, Sagging Skin.*

CUCUMBER TONIC

This tonic can be used for all skin types, but its toning and soothing properties are especially valuable for both dry and sensitive skins.

If possible, select a cucumber that has been organically grown and is free of pesticides. Wash the unpeeled cucumber and then chop it into large chunks. Process in a juice extractor, add the whole to an enamel or stainless steel pan and bring to the boil. Skim the juice, removing any scum, while it is being heated, then boil for five minutes. Remove from heat, cool, and allow to drip through filter paper. Add 1 part alcohol (vodka or brandy) to 2 parts juice. Stand for 12 hours, then filter until clear. Store in a tightly-sealed bottle. This tonic will last indefinitely.

Use this refreshing tonic each morning after washing your face. Soak a piece of cotton wool in the tonic and pat gently on your face.

Moisturising the Face

❖

Both cleansing and toning tend to dry facial skin slightly, removing some of the natural oils. A herbal moisturiser will replace these, keeping your skin supple and protecting it against moisture loss and external damage, dirt and grime.

AVOCADO MOISTURISING MASK

❖

Avocado oil is an excellent moisturiser to use under make-up, particularly in drying winds. Fresh avocado on the face and neck is especially nourishing for the skin.

Scoop out the flesh from half an avocado and mash into a pulp. Spread it on to the face and neck and lie down and relax for about 20 minutes while the oil of the fruit nourishes and moisturises your skin.

Remove with a piece of clean cloth, then dampened cotton wool.

MOISTURISER FOR YOUNG SKIN

❖

15 g (½ oz) beeswax
30 ml (1 fl oz) soya oil
35 ml (1 fl oz) almond oil
10 ml (⅓ fl oz) wheatgerm oil
10 ml (⅓ fl oz) aloe vera juice
30 ml (1 fl oz) lemon grass infusion
1 teaspoon clear honey
12 drops lemon juice
5 ml (⅙ fl oz) lemon grass oil
¼ teaspoon triethanalomine (optional)
3 drops tincture of benzoin

Melt the beeswax in a double pan over a medium heat. When completely liquid stir in the oils, aloe vera juice and lemon grass infusion, until well blended. Remove from heat, stir in honey. Pour into a ceramic bowl, add lemon juice, lemon grass oil, triethanalomine and tincture of benzoin, and beat until cool and of a creamy texture. Store in a sterilised glass jar with a tight-fitting lid.

Apply to face morning and night, rubbing gently into skin.

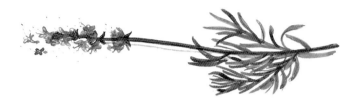

ANTI-WRINKLE MOISTURISER

Wrinkles are caused by inadequate skin care, through insufficient moisturising, and constant exposure to the elements, as well as by natural ageing. This results in dehydration, a weakening of the skin's ability to renew itself, and increasing rigidity of the collagen and elastin fibres.

Dehydration can be combated with an intensive care anti-wrinkle cream and a sensible approach to protecting the skin when outdoors in the sun.

This moisturiser is suitable for all skin types and will help to repair damaged skin.

25 g (1 oz) anhydrous lanolin
20 ml (⅔ fl oz) comfrey root water
25 ml (1 fl oz) avocado oil
25 ml (1 fl oz) almond oil
15 ml (½ fl oz) calendula oil
10 ml (⅓ fl oz) wheatgerm oil
10 ml (⅓ fl oz) witch hazel solution (from chemist)
10 ml (⅓ fl oz) aloe vera juice
¼ teaspoon triethanalomine (optional)
3 drops tincture of benzoin

Melt the lanolin with the comfrey root water in a double pan over a medium heat. When completely liquid stir in the oils, witch hazel solution and aloe vera juice, until well blended. Remove from heat, and pour into a ceramic bowl. Add the balance of ingredients and beat until cool and creamy. Store in a sterilised glass jar with a screw-top lid.
Gently massage a little cream into troubled areas each evening, or as needed.
TIP: Comfrey Root Water: Scrub and mince fresh comfrey root and steep in boiling water in a ceramic bowl for approximately three hours. Strain through muslin cloth and add required amount to the recipe. If you use dried root, simmer until soft.

ROSE MOISTURISING LOTION

A very light and gentle moisturiser suitable for all skin types.

40 ml (1½ fl oz) rosewater (from chemist)
30 ml (1 fl oz) glycerine
10 ml (⅓ fl oz) apricot kernel oil

Combine the ingredients in an amber-coloured glass bottle with a very tight-fitting lid, and shake well.

Acne

Although some acne is considered a teenage affliction, it can continue to be a problem beyond adolescence. It is a result of chronic inflammation of the sebaceous glands, causing thickened sebum, mixed with dead skin cells and grime, to block the mouth of the pores and form spots.

A good diet, incorporating plenty of fresh vegetables, fruit and wholegrain foods, and natural remedies will get your skin off to a good start and help to maintain a clear complexion. Remember, the benefits of cosmetic herbs and a good diet are cumulative.

HERBAL ACNE CREAM

This herbal ointment is an effective treatment for both teenage and adult acne.

20 g (⅔ oz) beeswax
40 ml (1½ fl oz) herbal water (see recipe following)
5 ml (⅙ fl oz) wheatgerm oil
2 teaspoons natural honey

Melt the beeswax in a double pan over low heat. When completely liquid stir in the herbal water and wheatgerm oil. Remove from heat and stir in the honey until thoroughly blended. Allow to cool, then store in a sterilised, screw-top glass jar. Apply to trouble spots morning and night, or as needed.

TIP: Herbal Water:
25 g (1 oz) marshmallow root, chopped
25 g (1 oz) malva leaf
500 ml (16 fl oz) distilled water

Put the herbs in an enamel or stainless steel pan and add distilled water. Bring to boil and then simmer for 30 minutes. Remove from heat, cover the pan, and allow to steep for 10 minutes. Strain through muslin cloth and add required quantity to recipe.

HERBAL TEA FOR ACNE
❖

In addition to using the acne preparations, a Malva and Marshmallow Tea should be taken morning and night whenever severe acne persists. To prepare, see Chapter Six.

A Sensible Routine to Help Control Acne

- Avoid too much stress — it can aggravate acne.
- Wash two or three times a day with soap formulated to deal with oily or acne skin. Instead of soap, cleanse with an acne herbal face scrub.
- Once a week deep cleanse with a herbal face mask.
- After cleansing your face apply a refining lotion.
- Treat troubled spots with a herbal acne cream.
- Don't pick at blemishes — you will spread them and leave scars.
- Make-up puffs, sponges or brushes that touch your face should be sterilised after each use or thrown out.
- Dirty make-up must go.
- Clean cotton wool is the best way to apply make-up. If you use an eyebrush, wash it in hot soapy water.
- Hair hanging over your face tends to aggravate acne.
- Ensure a good calcium intake. Dolomite in tablet form is excellent as it contains the correct balance of calcium and magnesium.

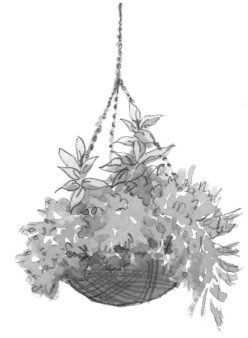

Oral Hygiene

❖

General mouth hygiene and the care of teeth and gums is just as important for natural beauty as is caring for skin and hair.

A well-balanced diet, which includes herbs that help to keep gums and teeth healthy, is essential. Healthy teeth need peak nutrition — especially the minerals, calcium, magnesium, phosphorus, and the trace elements. Herbs which provide these elements are:

Calcium	alfalfa, chamomile, dandelion, nettle, parsley, strawberry (fruit) and sunflower seeds
Magnesium	alfalfa, cayenne, dandelion, sunflower seeds and peppermint
Phosphorus	alfalfa, caraway, cayenne, chickweed, dandelion, garlic, kelp, parsley, sunflower seeds and watercress
Trace Minerals	alfalfa and kelp

Teeth

After brushing and rinsing, rub fresh sage leaves over your teeth and gums. This will leave your mouth feeling cleansed, and at the same time will whiten your teeth and strengthen your gums.

Herbal toothpastes are readily available, yet it is so simple and inexpensive to make your own tooth powder.

HERBAL TOOTHPOWDER

15 g (½ oz) fresh red sage leaves
10 g (⅓ oz) fresh peppermint leaves
25 g (1 oz) coarse sea salt

Mix the herbs and salt together and then spread them out on a baking tray. Place in a preheated oven 150°C (300°F) for 20 minutes, or until the herbs are crisp and dry. Pound the mixture with a pestle and mortar until reduced to a powder, then pass it through a fine sieve. Store in an airtight jar. To use, shake a little of the mixture into the palm of your hand and pick it up with a damp brush.

HERBAL BREATH FRESHENER

Sweet breath and a fresh-tasting mouth are as important as a complexion that glows with natural health.

2 teaspoons dried sage
1 teaspoon dried rosemary
1 teaspoon dried peppermint
500 ml (16 fl oz) boiling water
125 ml (4 fl oz) brandy or cider vinegar

Place all the herbs in a ceramic bowl and pour the boiling water over them. Add the brandy, or cider vinegar, and cover and steep for 2 hours. Strain through clean, sterile muslin, then drip through coffee filter paper, and store in an airtight bottle. Use as a soothing gargle or refreshing mouthwash as needed.

Beautiful Lips

Lips too suffer from the harshness of wind, sun and other elements, leaving them dry, chapped and cracked. Lips look and feel at their best when they are soft and smooth, and therefore need softening and protecting as regularly as the rest of your face.

A medicated and moisturising lip gloss will not only keep your lips moist and supple but will also soothe and repair them.

MEDICATED LIP GLOSS

10 g (⅓ oz) beeswax
5 g (⅙ oz) anhydrous lanolin
40 ml (1½ fl oz) wheatgerm oil
35 ml (1 fl oz) apricot oil
40 ml (1½ fl oz) rosemary infusion
5 drops essential oil of rosemary

Melt the beeswax and lanolin in a double pan over a medium heat. When completely liquid stir in the wheatgerm and apricot oils and rosemary infusion, until well blended. Remove from heat, pour into a ceramic bowl, add the rosemary oil and beat until cool. Store in a sterilised glass jar. Use as required.

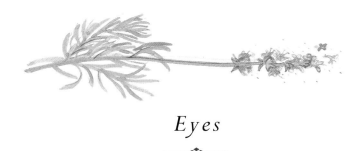

Eyes

❖

Eyes are the focal point of your face, and clear, sparkling eyes highlight the glow of a healthy complexion. To keep your eyes sparkling and beautiful they need plenty of sleep and relaxation, as well as a good mixed diet. To avoid tired, strained and bloodshot eyes:

- Make sure you take plenty of vitamin A (found in carrots and apricots).
- Sleep for eight hours a night as often as possible.
- Refrain from watching too much television.
- Don't read or use your eyes for close work in inadequate light.
- Refresh your eyes with a herbal eyebath if they have been exposed to a smoky atmosphere, salt water, excessive wind and sun.
- Bathe eyes with a soothing and healing herbal wash at the end of each day if you spend long hours working under artificial light.

Eye Lotions
TIRED, BLOODSHOT AND SORE EYES
❖

2 tablespoons fresh parsley
1 teaspoon dried elder flower
1 teaspoon fennel seed
300 ml (10 fl oz) boiling water

Place all ingredients in a ceramic bowl and pour water over them. Steep until the infusion becomes tepid, then strain through muslin cloth. Bathe eyes when required, using an eyebath.

Quick and Easy Eye Treatments

If you're feeling tired and your eyelids feel heavy, lie down in a quiet, semi-darkened room with your feet raised above the level of your head, and apply any of the following treatments:

Tea bags — squeeze out excess moisture and apply after they have cooled down.
Thin slices of raw potato — use for slight puffiness or a bruised sensation.
Slices of cucumber — cooling and soothing and will help to keep wrinkles at bay.

Day-to-Day Eye Care

The skin under the eye is very thin and delicate and care should be taken when removing make-up. Use a very fine oil, such as apricot or almond, to remove it so that it floats off.

After cleansing it is important to tone this tissue to ensure the skin retains its elasticity. Gently pat elder flower water on to surrounding eye tissue, avoiding an over generous application as this will only cause stinging.

ELDER FLOWER WATER

1 teaspoon dried elder flowers
300 ml (10 fl oz) boiling water

Place the herb in a ceramic bowl, cover with the boiling water and steep until cool. Strain through muslin cloth and bottle.

This infusion will last up to 7 days if kept in the refrigerator, provided its container has been sterilised. Check daily to ensure that it is still usable. You can extend the lotion's keeping qualities by adding 3–4 drops tincture of benzoin.

After toning, a light moisturising lotion should be dabbed on gently with the fingertips around the eye area. Never use heavy eye moisturising creams at night; they will leave your eyes baggy and puffy in the morning.

EYE MOISTURISING LOTION

30 ml (1 fl oz) apricot oil
30 ml (1 fl oz) almond oil
30 ml (1 fl oz) wheatgerm oil

Combine all the oils in a glass bottle with a tight-fitting lid and shake thoroughly to mix.

This lotion can be used anywhere on the face where lines are forming, and is best done last thing at night. The oils will be readily absorbed by the skin and help to plump out the lines.

Herbs for Healthy Hair

❖

The condition of your hair is usually a good indication of the state of your general health. And although diet is the foundation of healthy hair, herbs will also help to give it a natural beauty. To maintain that healthy lustre and body that is so important to your hair, try the gentle cleansing action of a herbal shampoo and conditioner. There is nothing more natural and refreshing than to wash your hair with a home-made herbal shampoo to keep it shiny, healthy and manageable.

However, unlike their commercial counterparts, shampoos made in the kitchen contain no synthetics, detergents or chemicals, in particular phosphates. They won't lather up like the store-bought variety, but they will leave your hair squeaky clean and in excellent condition.

Shampoos

Since there is so much variation in hair type, colour and texture, it is important to use the correct shampoo for your individual needs. For your particular requirements choose from those herbs listed below.

Shampoo Herbs

Fair Hair	chamomile — has a lightening effect and is healing to scalp irritations
Dark hair	rosemary or sage
Dandruff	nettle, parsley, peppermint, rosemary and thyme. Thyme, rosemary and peppermint combined not only control dandruff but act as a scalp and hair tonic.
Oily hair	sage, yarrow, rosemary and lime (linden) flowers
Healing	chamomile, parsley, rosemary and peppermint

The herbs are first prepared as an infusion, then added to a base recipe to make the shampoo.

Prepare the infusion by adding 3 tablespoons dried herbs to a ceramic bowl and covering with 2 litres (64 fl oz) boiling water. Cover, steep until cold, strain through muslin cloth, and add required quantity to the recipe.

BASE RECIPE

❖

100 g (3⅓ g) pure white soap, grated
juice of 1 lemon
1½ litres (48 fl oz) herbal infusion

Add the grated soap, lemon juice and 350 ml (12 fl oz) of the herbal infusion to a saucepan. Stir, and bring to the boil. Reduce heat and continue to stir until the soap has completely dissolved. Add the remaining herbal infusion, stirring until well blended. Bottle in a discarded shampoo bottle for future use.

You may choose from those herbs listed above, plus the following:

Normal hair	rosemary and sage for dark hair, chamomile and sage for fair hair, marigold (calendula) and alkanet for auburn hair
Dry hair	add elder flower or mallow to the infusion
Oily hair	those herbs listed for the soap-based shampoo, or a mixture of rosemary, lavender and yarrow. After shampooing, add 2 tablespoons of cider vinegar to the final rinsing water
Dandruff	choose from those herbs previously listed for the soap-based recipe

To prepare the infusion, add 2 tablespoons of your chosen herb, and 2 tablespoons dried soapwort, plus 1 litre (32 fl oz) water, to an enamel or stainless steel pan. Bring to the boil and then simmer for 15 minutes. Remove from heat, cover the pan, and allow to steep for 30 minutes. Strain through muslin cloth and add required amount to recipe.

OIL SHAMPOO

❖

An excellent shampoo that will not only cleanse but also help to moisturise and nourish. As in the previous shampoo, the herbs are first prepared as an infusion, then blended with the rest of the ingredients.

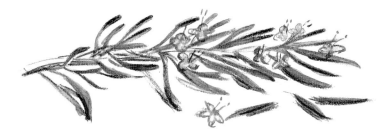

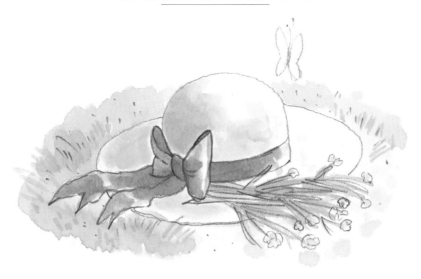

BASE RECIPE

30 ml (1 fl oz) almond oil
30 ml (1 fl oz) castor oil
180 ml (6 fl oz) herbal infusion

Combine all the ingredients in a suitable bottle, shake well, and store for future use. Shake before using.

Massage into scalp and hair for 1–2 minutes, then rinse thoroughly.

DRY SHAMPOO

When a busy schedule makes it impossible to wash your hair when it needs it the most, a dry shampoo is the answer.

15 g (½ oz) fuller's earth
4 drops essential oil of rosemary

Reduce the fuller's earth to a powder, mix in the rosemary oil and then pass the powder through a fine wire sieve.

Sprinkle a small amount over your hair and massage well in with your fingers. Leave for 10 minutes and then brush it out using a soft-bristle brush.

Conditioners

Your scalp, just like your facial skin, can dry out, leaving you with flaky skin and dandruff. This condition can be remedied by the regular use of a mildly antiseptic pre-wash conditioner that will stimulate, purify and moisturise your scalp. This conditioner has an almond oil base which is similar to your own scalp oil, and acts as an excellent emollient, protecting your skin by replacing natural surface oils.

ALMOND OIL CONDITIONER
❖
200 ml (6½ fl oz) almond oil
2 teaspoons dried peppermint
2 teaspoons dried rosemary
1 teaspoon fennel seed

Fill a suitable wide-mouthed jar with the almond oil and add the herbs. Seal tightly, and place where it will receive plenty of sunlight for at least 14 days, then strain and repeat the procedure with a fresh batch of herbs. Carefully strain the oil and store in an airtight, amber-coloured glass bottle.

Massage into your scalp whenever it needs extra conditioning or when dry and flaky skin is evident.

TIP: For dry hair that tangles when wet, pre-condition with a few drops of half rosemary oil and lavender oil. Massage well into scalp about half an hour before shampooing.

After Shampoo Conditioning Rinses

A conditioning rinse gives added health and shine to your hair. Use two or three times a week; it will help replace scalp oil lost through washing, remove shampoo residue, and balance the scalp's pH.

To make your rinse, place selected herbs in a ceramic bowl and pour boiling water over them. Steep overnight, strain through muslin cloth, and then add the lemon juice.

Store in a tightly-stoppered bottle in the refrigerator. After washing your hair, rinse it thoroughly with clean water and then pour over the herbal rinse.

Repeat several times, each time massaging well into your hair.

ANTI-DANDRUFF
❖
2 teaspoons dried rosemary
2 teaspoons dried thyme
1 teaspoon dried peppermint
2 tablespoons lemon juice
1 tablespoon dried chamomile for blonde hair or dried red sage for dark hair

Tips for Better Hair Care

Correct care of your hair is essential to keep its healthy lustre and bounce. The following tips will help you to maintain it in top condition:

- Wash your hair only when necessary; washing too frequently can overstimulate the scalp and leave you with dry, brittle ends.
- Use shampoo sparingly.
- Use a pre-wash conditioner before shampooing to take care of dry ends.
- Always wet hair thoroughly with warm water before applying shampoo. Very hot or very cold water are too much of a shock to the scalp.
- Rinse out all traces of shampoo and conditioner before drying your hair.
- After washing, dry your hair naturally. Pat the hair dry with a towel, and don't rub the hair or scalp hard.
- If it's a fine day, and you have the time, sit back and relax in the sun while you gently flick the moisture out with your fingertips, or loosely wrap it in a towel until it dries.
- Don't brush wet hair or you'll split the ends and pull it out by the roots.
- Use a very wide-toothed comb to gently comb out the hair.
- Never use a hair dryer, especially on dripping wet hair. If you must use one, towel dry first and then leave the dryer on a warm or cool setting.
- Excessive use of curling tongs and heated rollers will dry hair and make it brittle.
- Once a week, after shampooing, rinse your hair with 1 tablespoon of lemon juice diluted in 5 cups (1.25 litres/40 fl oz) water to restore the natural pH balance of your hair.
- Don't brush hair excessively or tease it; both will aggravate brittle, oily conditions. If you want to tease your hair, do it in sections starting at the roots.
- Don't use elastic bands to tie back hair or put it into plaits or a ponytail. They can cause hair to split. Use a covered band instead.
- Don't pull hair back tightly into a bun or ponytail. This will break your hair and cause it to split.
- Avoid using chemical bleaches and dyes — the chemicals in commercial colourants can cause skin irritation in some people, and even result in dermatitis. There are effective herbal alternatives.
- Avoid too many perms — they use too many chemicals. Often a good cut will do all that is needed for the body and shape of your hair.

- Before styling, dampen hair by using a pump-spray filled with water or herbal setting lotion. It will direct a controlled fine spray.
- Always keep brushes and combs spotlessly clean. Wash them in a diluted rosemary decoction (see Chapter Eight) to eliminate grease build-up.
- Have your hair cut about every six weeks to keep the style and get rid of split ends.
- After swimming in salt or chlorinated water, wash your hair with a herbal shampoo and then rinse with a chamomile rinse.
- Apply a chamomile rinse before you go swimming. As you swim it will slowly rinse away, protecting your hair from the harshness of chlorine and salt water.

Hair Colourants

There are simple and natural ways of colouring your hair using vegetable or herbal dyes. Unlike their synthetic, chemical counterparts, they are safer and kinder to your hair and scalp, and will not weaken or damage hair.

FAIR HAIR

To bring out blonde highlights or produce a gradual lightening effect over a long period.

2 tablespoons dried chamomile heads
500 ml (16 fl oz) boiling water

Add the herbs to a ceramic bowl, pour boiling water over and steep until cool. Strain through muslin cloth, and then repeatedly rinse your hair with the liquid after washing and rinsing the hair through with clear water.

Use after every shampoo.

DARK HAIR

To improve hair colour when it is showing signs of grey, or to darken fair hair, use the following dye.

1 tablespoon dried sage
1 tablespoon dried rosemary
500 ml (16 fl oz) boiling water

Prepare and use as for Fair Hair above.

AUBURN HAIR
❖

*Henna will give auburn highlights to fair hair and change its
colour to shades of red, or revive lost tones in auburn hair.*
4 tablespoons henna powder
boiling water and almond oil

Mix the powder with sufficient hot water to form a smooth paste. When
the mixture has cooled down, add a little almond oil and apply to the hair.
Cover with an old towel, aluminium foil and a shower cap to retain the
heat.

Leave for ½–2 hours before thoroughly rinsing out with clean water.

If you wish to tone down the redness, infuse sage in the boiling water
before mixing with the henna powder. To heighten the redness, replace the
sage with tea.

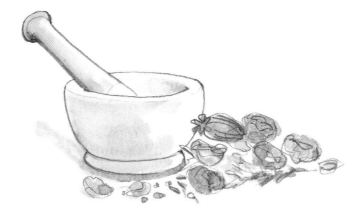

CHAPTER TWO
The Body Beautiful

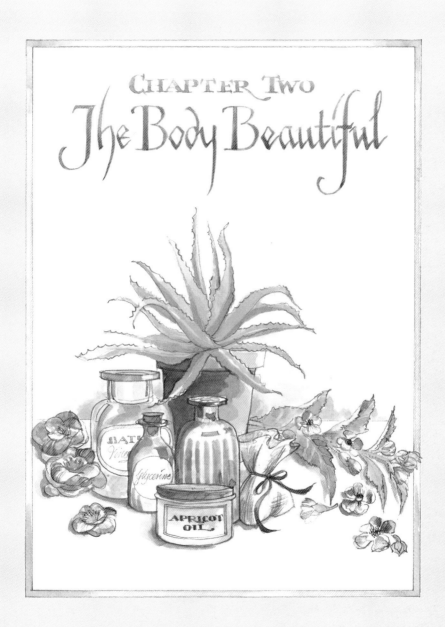

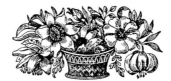

*M*any people lavish lots of attention on the care of their face, but neglect to give the same care to the rest of the body. A holistic approach to health and beauty requires that you maintain every part of yourself in the best possible condition.

Caring for your Hands

Your hands, like your face, are a focal point of your beauty and suffer harshly from the rigours of day-to-day living. Therefore they deserve special attention. They are affected by wind, sun, inclement weather, harsh cleaning agents and the many tasks which they are required to perform. This causes skin to become dry and scaly, or, in severe cases, chapped and split.

To keep them supple and looking beautiful, learn to protect them the natural way, with herbal softeners and moisturisers. And always follow the golden rules:

- Avoid direct contact with harsh detergents and cleansers, including washing-up liquid, scouring powders, and washing powder.
- Apply a protective barrier cream before commencing rough work, washing-up or messy household jobs.
- Use protective gloves for gardening, working on the car and other household chores as often as possible.
- Apply a nourishing hand cream morning and night, and immediately after any rough work or after washing.
- Wear natural fibre gloves when out of doors in cold weather.
- Use a natural skin repair cream whenever hands have suffered excessive exposure to salt water, sun, wind or other adverse climatic conditions; or when signs of roughening, chapping and cracking appear.

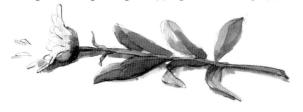

Hand Lotions
TOMATO HAND LOTION
❖

A quick and easy hand lotion to cleanse and soften the skin.

50 ml (1½ fl oz) tomato juice
50 ml (1½ fl oz) lemon juice
50 ml (1½ fl oz) glycerine

Mix together all ingredients in a bottle with a tight-fitting lid, and shake vigorously to ensure the lotion is well blended. Shake before use.

Massage well into hands and wrists.

OLD-FASHIONED LEMON HAND LOTION
❖

50 ml (1½ fl oz) lemon juice
50 ml (1½ fl oz) rosewater
50 ml (1½ fl oz) glycerine

Put all ingredients in a glass bottle, seal, and shake vigorously to mix.

This lotion will not only clean and nourish the hands, but will also strengthen the nails.

CALENDULA BARRIER CREAM
❖

Use this cream to protect your hands from drying detergents and grime. Smooth it into your hands before beginning rough work or immersing hands in soapy water.

2 tablespoons dried calendula flowers
1 cup (250 ml/8 fl oz) boiling water
30 ml (1 fl oz) almond oil
10 ml (⅓ fl oz) wheatgerm oil
2 teaspoons kaolin powder

Prepare an infusion of the calendula petals by steeping them in the boiling water. Cover, leave until cold, then strain through muslin cloth.

Mix 120 ml (⅔ fl oz) of the infusion with the rest of the ingredients until it forms a smooth cream. Store in a suitable glass jar.

Work well into hands. When the job is finished, wash hands with a gentle, pure soap, dry thoroughly and apply a hand cream or lotion.

Skin Repair

Often, due to excessive exposure to the elements, your hands or face can become chapped. To repair this damage a moisturiser is not always enough, so a soothing skin ointment should be used. The following lotion will help to alleviate both mild damage and severe chapping and cracking of the skin.

ELDER FLOWER LOTION
❖

50 ml (1½ fl oz) glycerine
50 ml (1½ fl oz) elder flower infusion
50 ml (1½ fl oz) aloe vera juice
25 ml (1 fl oz) wheatgerm oil
2 teaspoons lemon juice

Combine all the ingredients in a bottle, seal, then shake vigorously to mix. Shake well before using. Apply to affected areas of skin as needed.

Removing Stains

Blemished hands are unsightly and detract from your overall beauty. If your hands are spotted and stained after arduous housework or working in the garden, try a herbal stain remover.

LEMON AND BASIL
❖

juice of one lemon
fresh basil

Mix the lemon juice with a little basil and wash your hands with it. Let them dry naturally. Once dry, wash off the mixture.

If the stains have not completely disappeared, they will have faded somewhat and you can repeat the procedure the following day.

AGE SPOTS ON THE HANDS
❖

These large, freckle-like spots are usually part of the ageing process. However, lack of B-complex vitamins and vitamins E and C can worsen the problem. Increase your intake of these vitamins and rub the affected area with wheatgerm oil.

Healthy Fingernails

Most people subject their hands to a great deal of hard work, often resulting in tearing, splitting and chipping of the nails. Regular care is therefore essential, as is a healthy diet that provides calcium and a rich source of silica.

Helpful foods include barley, kelp, garlic, onion, parsley, rice, chives, celery, lettuce, borage flowers, sunflower seeds, and the herb 'horsetail' (*Equisetum arvense*). A regular nail bath and nail massage should also be included in your weekly health and beauty routine.

NAIL BATH

3 teaspoons dried horsetail
or
3 tablespoons fresh chives
3 teaspoons dried dill seed
300 ml (10 fl oz) boiling water

Put all the ingredients in a ceramic bowl and pour in the boiling water. Cover and allow to infuse overnight, then strain through muslin cloth. Store in a tightly-sealed jar in the refrigerator for up to 5 days.

Soak fingertips in the infusion morning and night for 15 minutes. Regular use of this nail bath will help to strengthen brittle nails. A herbal tea rich in silica should also be taken morning and night (see Chapter Six).

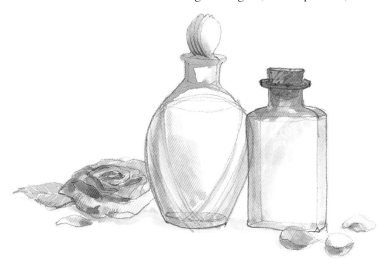

Caring for Arms and Legs

❖

Arms

Regular massage and exfoliation of the arms is essential. Massaging with a herbal lotion will improve the skin's elasticity and exfoliation with a loofah mitt or friction glove will improve circulation and rid the skin of dead, clogging cells.

If you don't have a loofah or friction mitt handy, you can exfoliate body skin by adding 2 tablespoons of medium oatmeal and 2 tablespoons of dried chamomile to a bath bag (see page 44). Oatmeal is a well-known skin softener, and as you rub your skin you will actually feel the impurities and rough skin float away.

The best time to exfoliate is when you're relaxing in an evening bath. After exfoliation, massage this herbal lotion into your skin:

80 ml (2½ fl oz) almond oil
40 ml (1½ fl oz) apricot oil
80 ml (2½) glycerine
20 ml (⅔ fl oz) aloe vera juice
1 teaspoon lemon juice
4 drops pumpkin oil
6 drops chamomile oil

Combine all ingredients in a suitable bottle with a tight-fitting lid, and shake until well blended. Store in a cool, dark place.

Use generously, massaging into the skin, moving from the wrists upwards. Maintain firm strokes, and keep massaging until all traces of the lotion have disappeared.

Elbows

Scrub elbows daily with a soapy pumice stone, or a bath bag filled with oatmeal, until all ingrained dirt has disappeared. Next, bleach the reddened skin with lemon juice and massage with any of the hand moisturising lotions and creams.

Legs

Thigh flab or cellulite are terms used to describe the ugly rippled bulges on the insides and backs of thighs. Swimming, dancing, cycling and yoga exercises are all ideal for keeping the leg muscles in trim.

Friction massage with a loofah or friction mitt during a warm bath is good for accelerating cell metabolism and improving the circulation. Coarse sea salt on the loofah helps to improve skin colour, and is excellent for clearing flaking skin and surface spots. Always massage upwards in the direction of the heart.

Lower legs also suffer from the same problems. As with the thighs, exfoliating with a loofah should be done several times a week at bathtime. Deal with more stubborn areas with coarse sea salt or an oatmeal bath bag; rinse off thoroughly, then massage with the following moisturising cream:

50 g (½ oz) anhydrous lanolin
50 ml (1½ fl oz) olive oil
25 ml (1 fl oz) apricot kernel oil

Melt the lanolin and oils together in a double pan over a low heat. Blend thoroughly, then pour the mixture into a suitable screw-top jar and allow to cool.

Massage into feet, legs and knees, smoothing it firmly upwards.

Caring for your Feet

At the end of a busy day most people like to relax and put their feet up. Yet there is nothing more soothing and relaxing than to put your feet down and soak them in an invigorating foot bath.

Reviving Tired Feet

At the end of the day revive tired feet by soaking them in a soothing foot bath. Then generously massage a soothing and healing foot oil into them.

SOOTHING FOOT BATH

2 tablespoons dried calendula petals
1 tablespoon dried lime flowers
1 tablespoon dried bay leaf
1 tablespoon sea salt

Place all the herbs in a bowl large enough for your feet and pour boiling water over them. Cover and allow to steep for 30 minutes, strain, discard herbs, and bring liquid to boil in a stainless steel or enamel pan. Pour the herbal water back into the bowl, stir in the sea salt until dissolved, leave to cool slightly and then soak your feet. After 10 minutes revive your feet with a quick dip into a basin of cold water, and then back again to the foot bath. Continue doing this as long as the hot water stays hot, then finish off with a cold dip.

Finish off by massaging into your feet the following lotion:

6 drops rosemary oil
15 ml (½ fl oz) almond oil
5 ml avocado oil

Blend the oils in a small, amber-coloured glass bottle and store in a cool, dark cupboard.

QUICK FOOT SOOTHER
❖

If you haven't time for a separate foot bath, rub diluted apple cider vinegar into your feet, massaging for about 5 minutes, before you take a bath.

Specific Foot Problems

If feet have been neglected or you suffer from corns, athlete's foot or any other specific problem, try the following natural remedies.

Persistent Soreness

Prepare as for the foot lotion but replace the rosemary with calendula (marigold) oil. Massage well into feet as required or after soaking.

Treating Corns

- Rub the corn every night with a crushed garlic clove, or put a sliver of garlic on the corn and hold it on with sticking plaster.
  Or,
- Apply freshly-crushed marigold leaves to the corn morning and night.

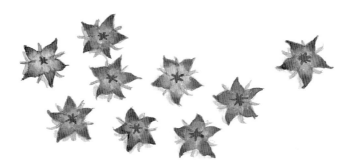

Athlete's Foot

This is characterised by soft, peeling skin between the toes, leaving your feet unusually clammy and quite often smelly. It is caused by a fungal infection which thrives where the acid balance of the skin has become too alkaline.

Athlete's foot is very infectious, so do not walk around barefoot where other people are likely to tread or allow the sharing of thongs, sandals or towels.

Wash your feet with soapwort decoction or apply poultices of red clover flowers (boiled first to soften them).

SOAPWORT DECOCTION
❖

40 g (1½ oz) dried soapwort root or leaves
1 litre (32 fl oz) distilled water

Put the herb and water in an enamel or stainless steel pan and boil for 30 minutes. Remove from heat, cover, allow to steep until cool, then strain through muslin cloth, squeezing all liquid from the herb. Store in a bottle with a pierced lid so that it can be squirted for ease of application.

After bathing feet, dry thoroughly with a towel that should be boiled after use. Rinse with diluted apple cider vinegar and dust lightly with this herbal foot powder between the toes when thoroughly dried.

HERBAL FOOT POWDER
❖

equal quantities of:
powdered orrisroot
powdered orange or lemon peel

Thinly pare the skin from the citrus fruit, making sure that no pith is left attached to it (otherwise the peel may go mouldy), and place in the sun until it is completely dry. Then place in a warm oven 100°C (212°F) until crisp. Remove and powder it in a blender or by rubbing through a fine wire sieve.

Mix thoroughly with the orrisroot powder and store in a container with holes punched in its lid.

Cold Feet

This is really a circulation problem and can be aided by plenty of exercise and sufficient vitamin E in your diet. Massaging with the following oil is also helpful:

6 drops essential oil of rosemary
15 ml (½ fl oz) almond oil
5 ml (⅙ fl oz) wheatgerm oil

Blend the oils thoroughly and store in an amber-coloured glass bottle in a cool spot. Use within 2 months.

Caring for your Body

❖

Keep your skin looking healthy and supple — herbal skin care preparations alone won't give your body that healthy glow. A holistic approach, which includes regular exercise and a good diet, is also essential to keep the body trim and the skin soft and supple.

Self-massage

Toning up with massage is an excellent supplement to a program of healthy exercise. It enhances relaxation, circulation, muscle tone and a general sense of wellbeing.

After bath, shower or exercise follow these simple steps:

- Pour a teaspoon of oil into your palm, rub your hands together, then apply to the breasts and buttocks with a circular motion.
- With a small amount of additional oil, rub your solar plexus six times in an anti-clockwise direction. Then stroke the residual oil upward on your stomach with both hands.
- Add another teaspoon of oil to your palm, rub your hands together and massage each arm with firm strokes from the hand to the shoulder. Finish off by deeply, yet gently, kneading up your arm with your fingers.
- Using one more teaspoon of oil, work upward on your legs with deep, firm strokes. Move from the ankle to the top of your thighs, working with both hands.

BODY MASSAGE OIL

selected essential oils
5 ml wheatgerm oil
5 ml avocado oil
40 ml (1½ fl oz) apricot kernel oil

Combine ingredients in a tightly-sealed, amber-coloured glass bottle. Shake vigorously until oils have emulsified. Label and date the bottle.

Selected Oils   Formulae (in drops)
   Normal skin   6 frankincense, 6 geranium, 3 jasmine, 12 lavender
   Dry skin   8 chamomile, 8 rose, 8 sandalwood
   Oily skin   8 cedarwood, 10 lemon, 6 ylang-ylang

THERAPEUTIC FOOT MASSAGE

Because your feet communicate with the rest of your body, a foot massage, combined with a therapeutic foot bath, will revive your entire system.

Before soaking your feet give each one a preliminary massage. Do this while sitting comfortably; place one foot over your knee and press, rub and pull each toe, then knead the sole with your knuckles. Next place the fingers of both hands on the sole, and the thumbs, pointing toward the toes, on the top of the foot, and stroke down from the ankles to the toes. Now put your feet in a foot bath and soak for 15 minutes.

Remove your feet, one at a time, drying them and then rubbing with the following massage oil:

24 drops calendula oil
5 ml (⅙ fl oz) wheatgerm oil
5 ml (⅙ fl oz) avocado oil
40 ml (1½ fl oz) almond oil

Combine all ingredients in an amber-coloured glass bottle and shake vigorously to blend them. Label and date the bottle.

Herbal Baths and Scrubs

Herbs added to the bath water not only provide a delightful fragrance, but will cleanse and soften your skin while you soak. They can be included as an infusion, in a bath bag, as essential oils or as a herbal vinegar.

The benefit of herbs may also be enjoyed in the shower, when your daily schedule doesn't allow for a relaxing bath. They are blended as fragrant and therapeutic body oil treats that whisk away the uppermost skin cells and soften and smooth your skin.

BATH BAG
❖

To make a bath bag, take a 20 cm (8 in) square of muslin, place the herbs in the centre, draw up the sides and tie with a piece of ribbon. Hang the bag from the tap under hot running water for maximum effect. Discard herbs after use — if you wish you may scrub your body with them first until the scent is completely exhausted.

The addition of a little dried soapwort will give the water a gentle cleansing effect.

WASH BAG
❖

Make the bag from a 25 cm square of muslin and tie with a drawstring or piece of ribbon. Fill with a mixture of equal parts oatmeal and dried herbs of your choice.

Gently scrub your body, paying particular attention to heels, knees and elbows. The oatmeal will cleanse and soften the skin and remove any dead cells. You will actually feel the impurities and rough skin floating away.

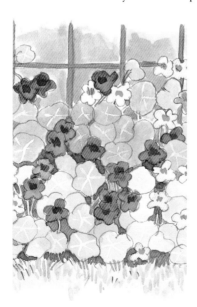

BATH OILS
❖

A fragrant bath oil can be made by using an odourless base oil, such as avocado, almond or sunflower. To make a bath oil dilute 30 drops of your chosen oil/s with 40 ml (1 1/2 fl oz) of base oil. Add about 10 drops of oil while the taps are running, and allow to stand for 5 minutes before bathing.

BATH VINEGAR
❖

Cider or wine vinegar added to the bath acts as an astringent, and will refresh and soften the skin. Bath vinegars are a better choice for those who have naturally greasy skin.

To make a herbal vinegar put 3 tablespoons of dried herbs (of your choice) into a large, wide-mouthed glass jar or ceramic pot. Heat together 250 ml (8 fl oz) each of vinegar and water to just below boiling point. Pour the heated liquid over the herbs, seal tightly, steep for 12 hours and strain. Add 1 cup (250 ml/8 fl oz) to the bath water while the taps are running.

Since bath vinegars will keep indefinitely, you can adjust the recipe to make a larger quantity, storing it in a tightly-sealed glass bottle ready for use.

Herbs to Choose From

To Invigorate and Rejuvenate: Rosemary, borage, lavender, nettle, valerian, peppermint, comfrey, yarrow, lovage and pine needles.

To Soothe Sore Skin: Comfrey, seaweed, marigold (calendula), woodruff, violets, Lady's mantle, marshmallow, chamomile and elder flowers.

To Ease Tired and Aching Muscles: Rosemary, bay leaf, honeysuckle, hyssop, angelica, lovage and chamomile.

To Relax, Soothe, Calm and Promote Sleep: Sage, lavender, rose petals, chamomile, lovage, lime (linden) flowers, elder flowers, pennyroyal, rosemary and yarrow.

To Comfort Tired and Frazzled Nerves: Pennyroyal, rosemary, bay leaf, chamomile, lime flowers and valerian.

To Refresh: Spearmint, lavender, lemon verbena and salad burnet.

To Sweeten Bath Water: Chamomile, rosemary, bay leaf and sage.

Salt Bath: A generous handful of sea salt is particularly beneficial if you have any broken or sore skin or scars to be healed.

OATMEAL BODY SCRUB

Gently massage into arms, legs, face and other parts of your body just prior to bathing. This scrub will exfoliate and soften skin and make it more receptive to any body oil applied after bathing.

100 g (3½ oz) of oatmeal
1 tablespoon chamomile infusion
3 tablespoons warm milk

Combine all ingredients, mixing thoroughly into a soft paste.

AROMATIC SHOWER
❖

Rub your entire body with a little bath oil containing stimulating or relaxing essences, diluted half-and-half with water. Put a plug in the shower drain and while showering sprinkle in the same aromatics, while the water collects. Your feet will benefit from the fragrant soak, while the ascending aroma will bring pure pleasure to your brain.

After-bath Care

To maintain that luxurious feeling of soft and smooth skin, an after-bath body lotion is essential. It will help to replace lost natural oils and moisturise at the same time.

HERBAL BODY POWDER
❖

An aromatic body powder is a delight to use after a bath or shower. Its mild deodorant properties and elusive scent will keep you feeling fresh and pampered.

90 g (3 oz) French chalk
50 g (1½ oz) cornflour
4 g magnesium carbonate
6 g calcium carbonate
1 tablespoon orrisroot powder
3 teaspoons lovage or rosemary infusion
1 teaspoon essential oil of choice

Mix the dry ingredients. Add the herbal infusion and essential oil and mix them through until the powder feels dry. Extra oil can be added if the scent is not strong enough, but take care not to get the mixture too wet. If it does become a little too wet adjust by adding more powder, a little at a time. Once dry, sieve twice through a fine wire sieve and store in a container with holes punched in its lid.

HERBAL DEODORANT
❖

Natural deodorants do not inhibit perspiration, but will control odours by preventing the growth of micro-organisms.

An effective deodorant can be made by steeping herbs in cider vinegar. It will have both a subdued perfume and antiseptic properties, and will keep you feeling fresh and odour free.

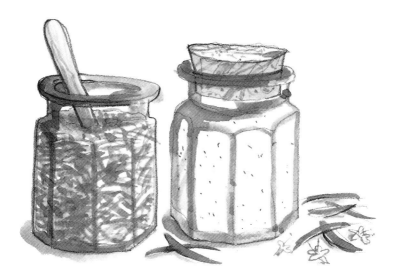

LIQUID DEODORANT

5 tablespoons fresh rosemary
4 tablespoons fresh lovage or thyme
cider vinegar

Place the herbs in a bowl, add a little cider vinegar and bruise the herbs with the back of a spoon. Put them in a large, wide-mouthed jar and pour over enough warmed vinegar to cover them. Tightly seal the jar and place where it will receive plenty of sunlight for 14 days. Strain through muslin cloth and dilute with distilled water: 2 tablespoons of water to 1 teaspoon of herb vinegar. Store in a well-sealed bottle.

After washing and drying under arms, dab on vinegar and allow to dry.

Other herbs suitable for deodorant vinegars: lavender, sage, scented geranium leaves, marjoram and honeysuckle.

Protection from the Sun

All of us like to spend time enjoying the open air, but having our skin exposed to too much sun will dry, burn or damage it. It is important therefore to limit your time in the sun and to take steps to prevent skin damage from arising.

To prevent premature ageing of the skin, wrinkles and the possibility of skin cancer, it is essential to wear a sunscreen, or keep covered up, when exposed to the sun.

AFTER-SUN MOISTURISER
❖

This moisturising lotion will assist in replenishing oils that have been lost through exposure to the sun.

30 ml (1 fl oz) rosewater
¼ teaspoon triethanalomine (optional)
50 ml (1½ fl oz) glycerine
20 ml (⅔ fl oz) aloe vera juice
10 ml (⅓ fl oz) peach kernel oil
10 ml (⅓ fl oz) wheatgerm oil
10 ml (⅓ fl oz) avocado oil
20 ml (⅔ fl oz) almond oil
6 drops essential oil of rosemary

Blend the rosewater and triethanalomine and thoroughly mix with the glycerine and aloe vera juice. Add the oils and beat continuously until the mixture emulsifies. Store in a tightly-sealed bottle in a cool, dark place.

Use generously, rubbing well into skin.

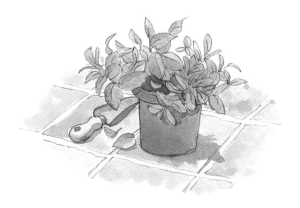

CHAPTER THREE
Herbs for Kids

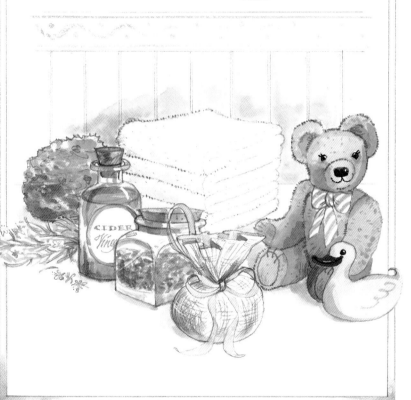

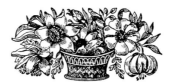

*H*ome-made herbal products for use at bathtime are a great way to introduce children to the many versatile uses of herbs for natural body care. It can give them a basic understanding of how and why we should work in harmony with nature and not against it. For it is important that our young ones realise, from an early age, that the natural things are the best, the purest, and the most beneficial.

Shampoos and Conditioners

❖

Choose from any of the herbs and recipes for hair care in Chapter One. For children who have a dandruff problem, rinse hair after washing with cider vinegar to restore the natural acid balance.

In cases of acne, add an infusion of malva, marshmallow and rosemary to the basic shampoo recipe. Use the following proportions:

25 g (1 oz) chopped marshmallow root
25 g (1 oz) malva leaf
2 litres (64 fl oz) distilled water
15 g (½ oz) rosemary leaf

Put the marshmallow and malva in a stainless steel or enamel pan and add the distilled water. Bring to the boil and then simmer for 30 minutes. Remove from heat, add rosemary, cover, and allow to steep until cool. Strain through muslin cloth, top up with distilled water, and add required amount to recipe.

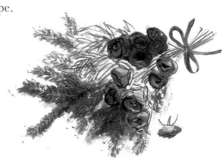

HAIR CONDITIONER OIL
❖

Use this for putting the lustre back into dry and lifeless hair.

equal quantities of:
olive, almond and avocado oil

Combine the oils and gently warm them to body temperature. Saturate the hair, then wrap it in a thick, hot towel and wait for 15 minutes before rinsing off.

Repeat weekly until no longer necessary.

Treating Head Lice

Severe itching of the head is the first sign of lice and nits. Thoroughly check the hair, looking close to the scalp — nits are grey-coloured eggs attached to the hair and are just visible with the naked eye. However, they are clearly visible with a magnifying glass.

An old-fashioned treatment is to use a hair rinse made from quassia chips. You will need:

15 g (½ oz) quassia chips
2 litres (64 fl oz) water
cider vinegar

Boil the chips for 2 hours, strain, and add 1 tablespoon of cider vinegar for every 300 ml (10 fl oz) of liquid.

Apply by combing through hair with a very fine comb. Repeat fortnightly, three times in all.

OIL TREATMENT
❖

25 drops rosemary oil
25 drops lavender oil
13 drops geranium (pelargonium) oil
12 drops eucalyptus oil
75 ml (2½ fl oz) almond oil

Combine all the oils in an egg cup, ensuring that they are well blended.

Divide the hair into small sections and saturate each section with the mixture down to the roots. Pile long hair on top of the head, ensuring that every bit is oiled.

Wrap plastic around the head and behind the ears to stop the oils from evaporating. Make sure that small children cannot move the plastic anywhere near the nose or mouth and restrict breathing.

Leave on for 2 hours, remove and shampoo, rubbing in well. Rinse thoroughly and comb through with a fine comb. Repeat 3 days later.

For the Bath

❖

SOAPY WASH BAG
❖

Great for scrubbing the kids clean and softening the skin at the same time. Make the bag from a 25 cm (10 in) square of muslin and attach a drawstring to close it.

Mix together 2 tablespoons of dried herbs (choose from those listed on page 45, Herbal Baths), 2 tablespoons of medium oatmeal, and 1 tablespoon of pure, unscented, grated white soap. Place the mixture in the bag and use to gently wash the body.

SCENTED BATH SALTS
❖

This is the herbal mixture my teenage daughter adds to the bath when she feels the need to luxuriate. You will need the following:

560 g (18 oz) bicarbonate of soda
15 g (½ oz) dried lavender
8 ml (⅓ fl oz) oil of rosemary
8 ml (½ fl oz) eucalyptus oil

Thoroughly mix all ingredients and store in a jar with a tight-fitting lid.

To use, add a couple of handfuls to a square of muslin, draw up the sides and tie with a piece of ribbon. Swirl around in the bath water and leave in the bag. When you've finished soaking, rub the muslin bag over your body until the scent of the lavender is exhausted.

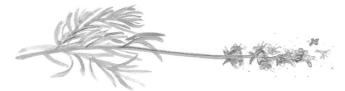

SOAP BUBBLE LIQUID

This is a great way for kids to enjoy their bath, at the same time washing away dirt and grime.

aromatic dried herb of choice
40 parts soft water
2 parts grated pure white soap
30 parts glycerine

Put the dried herb — in the proportion of 2 teaspoons to every 300 ml of boiling water — in a ceramic bowl and add the soft water. Cover, steep overnight and strain through muslin cloth.

Hard water can be softened by adding either washing soda or bicarbonate of soda in the following proportion: 45 g (1½ oz) to every 4 litres (128 fl oz) of water.

Place the grated soap and herb water in an enamel pan and dissolve together over a medium heat, stirring continuously. Stir in the glycerine until well blended. Remove from heat, cool, and store in a tightly-capped bottle.

Pour a small amount into the bath while the taps are running, and swish around to create the bubbles.

SOAPWORT SHOWER GEL

This is a gentle cleansing gel ideal for older children and teenagers who prefer to use it in the shower.

40 g (1½ oz) dried soapwort root or leaves
600 ml (20 fl oz) water
15 ml (½ fl oz) vodka
powdered arrowroot

Put the herb and water in an enamel pan and bring to the boil; allow to boil for 4 minutes. Remove from heat, cover and steep for 30 minutes. Strain through muslin, measure the liquid, return to the pan. Add the vodka, and 2 teaspoons of powdered arrowroot to every 80 ml (2½ fl oz) of liquid. Heat gently, stirring continuously until the mixture thickens and clears. Remove from heat and store in a wide-mouthed container.

Rub the gel over your body while showering for a gentle cleansing effect that leaves the skin soft and smooth.

Skin Care

T O N E R   F O R   Y O U N G   H E A L T H Y   S K I N

This tonic will redress the skin's pH balance and remove the last traces of grease, dead skin cells and grime.

1 teaspoon dried chamomile
2 teaspoons dried rose petals
2 teaspoons dried thyme
3 tablespoons fresh mint

C L E A N S I N G   M A S K   F O R   L A R G E   P O R E S

4 cups fresh sage leaves
1 teaspoon fennel seeds
2 teaspoons fennel leaves

Place the herbs in a pan and cover with boiling water. Simmer for about 10 minutes or until the herbs combine into a thick mash, then set aside to cool. Spread mash, while still warm, over a piece of sterile cotton or lint and apply to your face, avoiding eyes and mouth. Leave for 15 minutes, then wash off with lukewarm water, rinsing well. Splash the skin with cold water and pat dry with a soft towel.

A C N E   F A C E   S C R U B

4 tablespoons fuller's earth
2 tablespoons oatmeal
4 tablespoons finely ground thyme and chickweed, or lemon grass
1 tablespoon ground fennel seed
12 drops lemon juice
aloe vera juice
almond oil
natural yoghurt
1½ tablespoons brewer's yeast
2 teaspoons natural honey

Mix together all ingredients, adding sufficient yoghurt, oil and aloe vera juice to form a thick paste. Apply to your face and neck, avoiding the area

around the eyes and any broken skin. Massage lightly into your skin for 5
or 6 minutes and then remove by rinsing thoroughly.

Apply a refining lotion, followed by a moisturising cream, after your
shower.

Oral Hygiene

SPEARMINT MOUTHWASH

❖

*A pleasant-tasting mouthwash which helps to keep the gums in
a healthy condition.*

125 ml (4 fl oz) vodka or brandy
30 g powdered myrrh
spearmint oil
125 ml (4 fl oz) distilled water

Put the vodka or brandy in a glass jar, add the myrrh, seal and allow to
stand for 14 days, shaking daily. Strain through coffee filter paper, add a
few drops of spearmint oil, and dilute with the distilled water. Store in a
glass bottle with a tight-fitting lid.

Use to rinse out the mouth as needed.

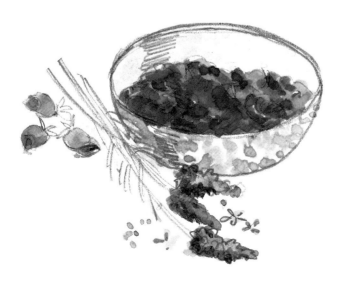

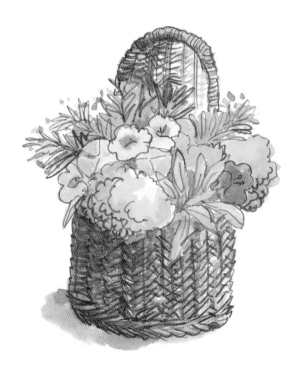

CHAPTER FOUR
Just for Men

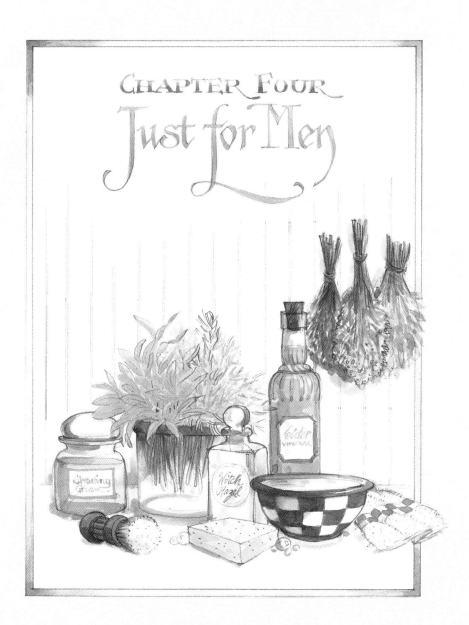

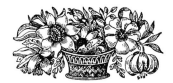

*V*ery seldom are men considered when it comes to natural skin care and home-made herbal products. Yet bit by bit, men who were once cool as cucumbers are warming to the concept of facial skin care. Today's man is starting to take care of his skin, hair, hands and nails.

While all the recipes in this book may be used by men and women alike, this chapter is specially for men.

Fortnightly Facial Routine

❖

Follow this simple five-step routine once every two weeks to keep facial skin in sparkling condition.

Step 1: Cleanse

Wash your face with the Chamomile Soap in Chapter Five, or, if your skin is very sensitive, use the Lavender Cleansing Lotion on page 15. Massage into skin and remove with a damp cotton wool ball until all grime disappears.

Step 2: Deep Cleanse

Steam your face by putting it over a bowl of hot water for no longer than 10 minutes with a towel forming a tent over your head. Add 20 drops of essential oil of lavender or eucalyptus to 1 litre (32 fl oz) water, to enhance the cleansing effect. Or use the Oatmeal Face Scrub or a face mask suitable to your skin type from Chapter One.

Step 3: Shave

Work up a good lather with a shaving soap or cream, so that the skin does not dry out. Soften up the beard by using a brush, then shave using downward strokes; shaving upwards cuts into the skin. Use small strokes on sensitive skin such as the cheeks and upper lip. Shave the areas of tougher skin last.

Step 4: Tone

Instead of patting freshly shaved skin with a commercial aftershave, use a herbal aftershave lotion to tone your skin. Commercial aftershaves contain a high percentage of alcohol, which stings the pores. Herbal toners act as gentle antiseptics that close the pores and condition the skin.

Step 5: Moisturise

Finish off the routine by massaging the face and neck with a light moisturiser. Massaging the skin is also good for the circulation.

If facial skin feels dry after shaving and toning, lightly dab with apricot kernel oil. This oil can also be used for your day-to-day shaving routine.

Beards and Moustaches

Beards and moustaches also require attention and regular grooming. Wash them every time you wash your face, using the fingertips to massage the skin underneath. Dry, then apply a herbal oil such as basil, rosemary or sage.

To apply the oil, rub a little of it between the palms of the hand and stroke a good quality hairbrush over them to pick up the oil. Brush through the beard and moustache — if the latter is too difficult use a toothbrush.

SHAVING SOAP

This recipe makes a subtly fragrant soap, ideal for shaving with.

1 cake non-scented, pure white soap, grated
distilled water
4 drops essential oil of lavender
2 drops essential oil of thyme
1 drop essential oil of peppermint
5 drops essential oil of bergamot

Melt soap in an enamel pan, over a low heat, with enough distilled water to form a soft paste (use a potato masher to help dissolve soap). Stir in essential oils until well blended, remove from heat and spoon into a wide-mouthed, shallow container. Let soap harden for 48 hours before use.

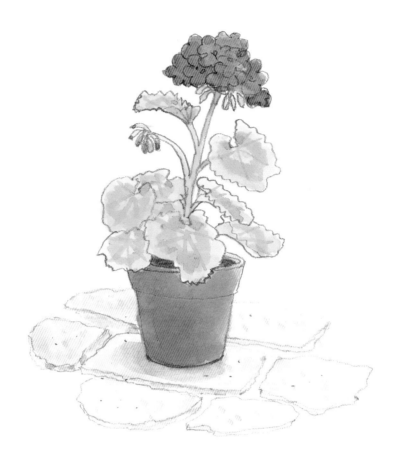

SHAVING CREAM

❖

*This soft cream is excellent for those who prefer not to use a
shaving brush and lather up.*

½ cake non-scented, pure white soap, grated
distilled water
175 ml (⅙ fl oz) rosewater
175 ml (⅙ fl oz) vodka

Melt the soap in an enamel pan, over a low heat, with just enough distilled
water to form a soft paste when cold. Dissolve rosewater in alcohol and
mix with soap paste. Store in a wide-mouthed, screw-top jar.

Apply to face with fingers, and smooth over beard.

Skin Care

❖

HERBAL AFTERSHAVE TONING LOTION

1½ tablespoons chopped sage leaves
1½ tablespoons rosemary leaves
1½ cups (375 ml/12 fl oz) cider vinegar
1½ cups (375 ml/12 fl oz) witch hazel (from the chemist)

Put the herbs in a large glass jar and pour in warmed cider vinegar. Seal tightly and leave to steep for one week, in a place where it will receive plenty of hot sun — a sunny windowsill is ideal. Strain the liquid off and add it to the witch hazel, stirring until well blended. Store in a tightly-capped bottle. Pat on to skin after shaving.

FACIAL MUSCLE TONER

Areas of flabby facial muscle can be firmed up with the aid of this toner.

handful ivy leaves
boiling water

Finely chop ivy leaves and boil in a little water for 10 to 15 minutes, until mixture is the consistency of a thick mash (make sure the infusion does not boil dry), then set aside to cool a little. Apply (while still warm) with pieces of sterile lint or cotton wool. Leave on for 15 minutes and then wash off with lukewarm water, rinsing well. Splash skin with cold water, and pat dry with a soft towel.

ROSEWATER LOTION

❖

An ideal moisturiser for normal skin. Apply immediately after shaving and toning.

¼ teaspoon triethanalomine (optional)
180 ml (6 fl oz) rosewater
40 ml (1½ fl oz) almond oil
20 ml (⅔ fl oz) glycerine
10 ml (⅓ fl oz) witch hazel

Dissolve the triethanalomine in the rosewater, then add the rest of the ingredients and beat until the mixture emulsifies. Store in a suitable bottle.

Apply to face and neck and gently massage in with your fingertips.

LEMON MOISTURISING LOTION

❖

An ideal moisturising lotion for oily skin, this helps to control overactive sebaceous glands as well as correcting the skin's pH balance.

¼ teaspoon triethanalomine (optional)
60 ml (2 fl oz) rosewater
40 ml (1½ fl oz) almond oil
20 ml (⅔ fl oz) glycerine
40 ml (1½ fl oz) witch hazel
40 ml (1½ fl oz) freshly strained lemon juice

Prepare as for *Rosewater Lotion.*

COMBINATION SKIN MOISTURISER

❖

Apply the *Lemon Moisturising Lotion* to the centre panel of the face, and the *Rosewater Lotion* to the rest of the skin.

PRE-SHOWER BODY SCRUB

❖

To use, gently massage handfuls of this mixture into arms, legs, face and other parts of your body just before bathing. This scrub will exfoliate and soften skin and make it more receptive to any body oil applied after bathing.

4 tablespoons fine table salt
1 very ripe avocado
3 drops essential oil of neroli

Thoroughly mix all ingredients in a ceramic bowl.

REFRESHING BODY COLOGNE

❖

This is ideal to use on hot summer days or nights. It has a tangy lemon scent and will leave you feeling fresh and cool.

22 drops essential oil of lemon grass
125 drops essential oil of lemon peel
30 drops essential oil of neroli
250 ml (8 fl oz) vodka

Mix all the ingredients thoroughly and allow the mixture to stand for a month. Drip through filter paper and store in a tightly-sealed bottle.

BODY POWDER

❖

A slightly aromatic body powder with mild deodorant properties to use after a bath or shower.

90 g (3 oz) French chalk
50 g (1½ oz) cornflour
4 g magnesium carbonate
6 g calcium carbonate
1 tablespoon orrisroot powder
25 drops essential oil of thyme
13 drops essential oil of peppermint
62 drops essential oil of bergamot
3 teaspoons lovage infusion

Mix the dry ingredients. Add the essential oils and herbal infusion and mix them through until the powder feels dry. If the mixture is too wet or not sufficiently scented, adjust by adding more powder or essential oil, a little at a time. Once dry, sieve twice through a fine wire sieve and store in a container with holes in its lid.

Other herbs suitable for the infusion: marjoram, sage and rosemary.

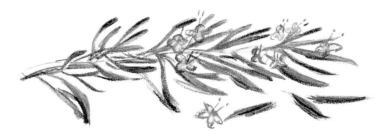

SOYA MEAL MASK AND TONIC
❖

A cleansing mask suitable for all skin types, that will also nourish and revitalise tired skin.

3 tablespoons soya meal
2 teaspoons ground alfalfa seeds
2 teaspoons dried chamomile, ground
2 teaspoons dried rose leaves, ground
wheatgerm oil and warm water

Mix together all ingredients, add a little warm water and sufficient oil to make a paste, and apply to the face and neck. Leave for 15 minutes, then wash off with lukewarm water.

Oral Hygiene

SAGE MOUTHWASH AND GARGLE
❖

1 cup (250 ml/8 fl oz) milk
1 tablespoon fresh sage leaves
or
2 teaspoons dried sage

Combine chopped sage with milk and bring to simmering point in a covered saucepan. Remove from heat, cool, strain and use as needed.

CHAPTER FIVE
Skin Deep

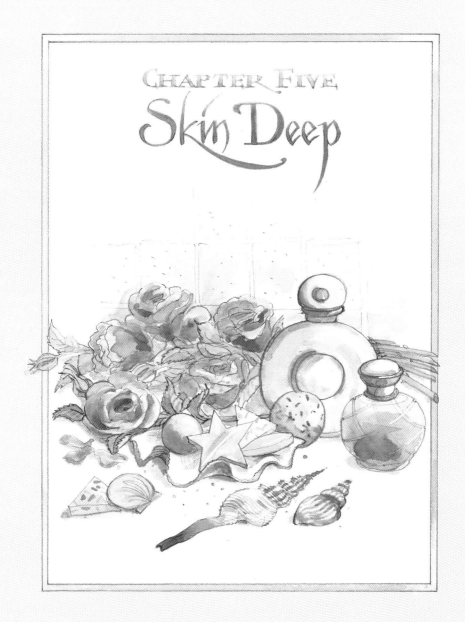

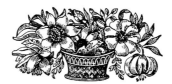

A good herbal soap exerts its effects on the outer layer of the skin — the so-called horny or epithelial layer — making it smooth and soft. Since basic skin care begins with cleansing, an ideal way to gain full value from the use of herbs is to include them in making your own soap, which will rinse away dirt and smooth the skin.

Cleansing the Skin

❖

CHAMOMILE SOAP

❖

A gentle soap that is suitable for all skin types, including disturbed skin, and is both soothing and healing.

5 tablespoons dried chamomile
300 ml (10 fl oz) boiling water
350 g (12 oz) pure, unscented soap, grated

Place the herb in a ceramic bowl and add the boiling water. Cover, infuse for 12 hours, strain through muslin, squeezing all liquid from the herbs, and add to recipe.

Melt the grated soap in an enamel pan over a low heat with just enough of the chamomile infusion to form a soft paste (use a potato masher to help dissolve soap). Add the remaining infusion and stir continuously until thoroughly blended. Remove from heat and pour into suitable moulds.

Moulds for the soap mixture can be small, shallow cardboard boxes, patty pans, chocolate moulds, circles, triangles, etc — anything you can think of. Allow to harden, remove from moulds, and it is ready for use.

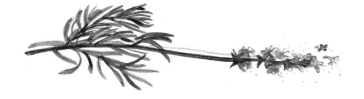

YARROW SOAP

An excellent soap for oily skin and overactive sebaceous glands.

3 tablespoons dried yarrow
300 ml (10 fl oz) boiling water
350 g (12 oz) pure, unscented, grated soap

Prepare as for *Chamomile Soap.*

COSMETIC HERB SOAP

❖

A good one to use on oily, problem skin, and where there are blackheads.

450 g (15 oz) pure, unscented, grated soap
250 ml (8 fl oz) lavender infusion
purified borax
225 g (7½ oz) almond meal

Add the grated soap and lavender infusion to an enamel pan and melt over a medium heat. To this mixture add borax — in the proportion of 1 part to 10 by volume — and almond meal. Mix well by stirring for about 10 minutes. Remove from heat and pour into a large, shallow tray lined with damp muslin. Allow to cool then cut into cakes. Ready to use immediately.

CALENDULA SOAP

❖

Use this whenever you need a medicated soap.

25 g (1 oz) chopped marshmallow root
25 g (1 oz) malva leaf
1 litre (35 fl oz) distilled water
5 tablespoons dried calendula petals
350 g (12 oz) pure, unscented, grated soap

Put the marshmallow and malva in an enamel or stainless steel pan and add distilled water. Bring to the boil and then boil gently for 30 minutes. Remove from heat, add the calendula petals, cover, and allow to steep for 8 hours. Strain through muslin and add required amount to recipe.

Melt grated soap over low heat with 300 ml (10 fl oz) of the herbal infusion. Stir continuously until soap has completely dissolved — use a potato masher to help dissolve it. Remove from heat and pour into suitable moulds. Allow to harden, remove from moulds, and it is ready for use.

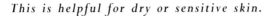

H O N E Y   S O A P

❖

This is helpful for dry or sensitive skin.

900 g (30 oz) pure, unscented, grated soap
elder flower infusion
110 g (4 oz) unprocessed honey
110 g (4 oz) almond oil
110 g (4 oz) purified borax

Put the grated soap in the top of a double boiler with barely enough hot elder flower infusion to cover. Melt over boiling water, stir thoroughly and add the honey, almond oil and borax. Mix well by continuing to stir for about 10 minutes, then add a few drops of any preferred essential oil for scent, and remove from heat. Pour liquid soap into a large, shallow tray lined with damp muslin and allow to cool. When it has hardened, cut into cakes and it is ready for use.

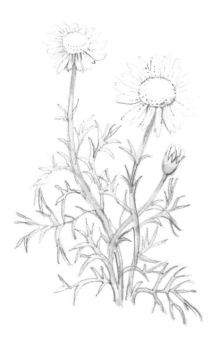

O A T M E A L   S O A P

❖

Oatmeal is soothing and healing to the skin, and when included in soap will exfoliate and soften it. Suitable for all skin types.

Prepare as you would the Cosmetic Herb Soap, replacing the lavender infusion with chamomile.

FLORAL WASHBALLS
❖

300 g (10 oz) pure, unscented soap
300 ml (10 fl oz) rosewater
10 drops oil of cloves
3 tablespoons dried lavender flowers
3 tablespoons dried rose petals
2 tablespoons dried sweet marjoram

Grate the soap into a large ceramic mixing bowl. Heat 250 ml (8 fl oz) of rosewater to just below boiling point and pour it over the soap. Blend thoroughly, using a wooden spoon, and allow to stand for 10 minutes. Knead with your hands to make a smooth paste, and mix in the oil of cloves, lavender flowers, rose petals and marjoram. Leave in a warm spot for 10 minutes or until the mixture begins to dry and become pliable. Form the soap into small balls, about the size of a golf ball, and leave to firm up in the sun, on a sheet of plastic film, for about 2 hours.

Moisten your hands with the remaining rosewater and rub the balls to make them smooth and shiny, then place them back on the plastic film and leave in a warm spot for 24 hours to firm completely.

SOAPWORT BATHING LIQUID
❖

40 g (1½ oz) dried soapwort root or leaves
1 litre (32 fl oz) water
20 g (⅔ oz) dried rosemary leaves

Put the soapwort and water in an enamel pan and boil for 20 minutes. Remove from heat, add rosemary, cover, and steep overnight. Strain through muslin, squeezing any remaining liquid from the herbs, and store in a tightly-sealed bottle in a cool place.

Half a cup (125 ml/4 fl oz) of liquid added to the bath water will give it a gentle cleansing effect that leaves the skin feeling smooth and soft, as well as stimulating the circulation and relaxing aching muscles.

OATMEAL SANDSOAP

Keep this in the laundry and use after working around the yard or in the workshop. It will clean the dirtiest hands, removing ingrained stains and grease.

purified borax
soap scraps
glycerine
medium oatmeal
sifted, clean white sand

Make a saturated solution of borax in 500 ml (16 fl oz) water, and cut or grate into it any bits and pieces of soap. Add 25 ml (1 fl oz) of glycerine and let the mixture boil until the soap is dissolved and is as thick as cream. If it is not thick enough, add more soap, or if it is too thick add more water, a little at a time.

Stir in sufficient oatmeal and white sand, a bit at a time, to make a soft paste, and pour into a shallow mould lined with damp muslin. Allow to harden and cut into cakes.

LEMON VERBENA CREAM CLEANSER

If you prefer to use a cleansing lotion to a soap, this recipe is excellent for removing city grime and stale make-up.

15 g (½ oz) beeswax
55 ml (2 fl oz) almond oil
10 ml (½ fl oz) avocado oil
10 ml (½ fl oz) wheatgerm oil
40 ml (1½ fl oz) lemon verbena infusion (see Chapter Eight)
¼ teaspoon triethanalomine (optional)

Melt the wax in a double pan over low heat. When completely liquid, stir in the oils and infusion until well blended. Remove from heat, pour into a ceramic bowl, add triethanalomine and stir vigorously until cool and of a creamy texture. Store in a sterilised screwtop glass jar.

Apply a small amount to facial skin morning and night, massaging in gently, and then remove all traces with a soft piece of clean cloth.

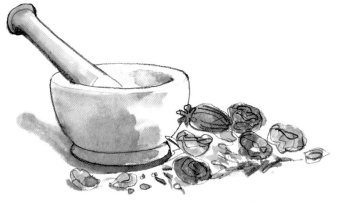

Toning the Skin

❖

REFINING LOTION

❖

If you suffer from acne, skin eruptions or problem skin, a refining lotion should be used immediately after cleansing facial skin.

2 teaspoons dried calendula flowers
1 teaspoon dried chamomile
1 teaspoon dried thyme
1 teaspoon dried, chopped lemon grass
500 ml (16 fl oz) white wine vinegar

Put the herbs into a large, wide-necked jar that has an airtight stopper. Gently warm the wine vinegar and pour over the herbs. Seal the jar and leave in a sunny location for about 2 weeks. Shake the contents every day and then test at the end of the 14 days by placing a little vinegar on the back of your hand. If it doesn't smell strongly of the herbs, repeat the procedure with a fresh batch of herbs.

Strain through muslin cloth and store in a tightly-sealed bottle.

To use, mix 1 tablespoon of the herbal vinegar with 150 ml(5 fl oz) of distilled water. Apply immediately after cleansing facial skin by dabbing the lotion onto problem areas with a piece of sterile cloth.

Use a cleansing lotion or cream, rather than soap, prior to applying this refining lotion, as vinegar decomposes soap residue.

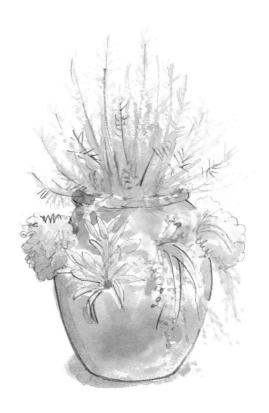

CHAPTER SIX
Beauty from Within

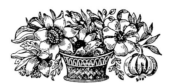

*B*eauty is not only skin deep — true beauty radiates from within, and to maintain that healthy glow to your complexion it is important to ensure that the internal body systems are functioning in tip-top condition. Herbal teas aid in this task and, if drunk regularly, will have a beneficial effect, as well as clearing the complexion.

Herbal teas are simple and easy to make. Most ingredients are readily available from specialty shops, such as health food or herbal gift shops. However, it is best to either grow your own herbs or gather them from a safe and reliable source, so that they can be used fresh or dried and stored in suitable screw-top glass jars.

You can drink herbal teas alone or blended for additional beneficial effects: they are the gentle way to good health!

General Directions

- Unless specific directions are given for a recipe, a herbal tea is made by infusing the herb in the following proportions:
  1 tablespoon fresh herb or 1 level teaspoon dried herb to 300 ml (10 fl oz) boiling water
  For individual cups, pour in the hot water, cover, infuse for 3 minutes, and strain into another cup.
  If brewing in a teapot, allow 1 serve per individual and 1 for the pot. Infuse for 5 minutes in boiling water, then strain into individual cups.
- Bark and root will not yield their properties to an infusion. Prepare these as a decoction — see Chapter Eight.
- A tea can be drunk at any time during the day, and with the addition of honey, a slice of lemon, or a tablespoon of orange flower water or rosewater.
- When making a flower tea modify the procedure as follows:
  first bring the measured amount of water to boil in an enamel or stainless steel saucepan. Add the flowers, replace the lid, and simmer for 1 minute. Remove from heat and allow to infuse for 3 minutes, then strain into individual cups.
- Any excess tea made in the morning can be stored in the refrigerator for use later in the day.
- In summer, teas can be chilled in the refrigerator and drunk with the addition of ice and mineral water or fresh fruit juice.

Herbal Drinks

❖

STRENGTHENING FINGERNAILS

❖

3 tablespoons fresh borage flowers
or
1 teaspoon dried herb
3 tablespoons fresh chives
or
1 teaspoon dried horsetail
500 ml (16 fl oz) boiling water

Put the herbs in a ceramic teapot, add boiling water, infuse for 7 minutes, then strain into a cup. Drink one cup morning and night, or as needed, but not more than four cups a day.

To speed up the beneficial effect and power of the tea add a pinch of cayenne.

If substituting the horsetail for the chives, make the tea by the following method: Put the horsetail in an enamel pan, bring to the boil, and then simmer for 30 minutes. Remove from heat, add borage flowers and steep for 15 minutes. Strain into a cup.

SUBSTITUTE FOR CHINA OR INDIAN TEA

❖

Unlike China or Indian teas, natural herbal blends contain no caffeine or tannin, both very strong stimulants. The following recipe is an ideal introduction to herbal teas, especially for those people who are used to drinking ordinary tea.

dried red clover
dried dandelion leaf
dried peppermint leaf

Blend equal parts of all three herbs and store in a screw-top glass jar.

Coffee Substitute

Coffee, like traditional tea, is high in caffeine and adversely affects the body systems.

For coffee drinkers the following herbal substitute will not only provide a healthy alternative, but will act as a general tonic to fortify the body systems.

DANDELION COFFEE

❖

Wash and dry the roots and cut into rings about 2 cm (¾ in) thick. Roast the pieces of dandelion root in a hot oven (200°C/475°F) for 20 minutes, then reduce to granules in a coffee bean grinder or blender. Use in the same way as instant coffee.

Herbal Teas

Herb	Parts Used	Application and Effect
angelica	leaf	for headaches and exhaustion; acts as a general tonic and soothes the nerves; digestive
anise	seed	sweetens the breath and refreshes the palate; for diarrhoea and indigestion; soothing
balm (lemon)	leaf	relaxing, refreshing, soothing
basil	leaf	for gastric upsets and colds; acts as a tonic that strengthens the body systems
blackberry	whole plant	clears up minor skin disorders
borage	flower	for catarrh; stimulant, diuretic, exhilarating; aids in the healthy growth of hair and nails
caraway	seed	helpful in clearing the complexion
chamomile	flowers	for sore throat, mouth infections (as a gargle); digestive, soothing; will help to induce sound natural sleep
chervil	leaf	said to brighten dull eyes and clear the complexion
chicory	flower	reputed to give skin a healthy glow; use in moderation
chives	leaf	will help to strengthen nails and teeth
cayenne	fruit	used in conjunction with other herbs it acts as a catalyst, increasing their power and speeding up their beneficial effect

Herb	Parts Used	Application and Effect
coriander	seed	traditionally used for purifying the blood, thus clearing the complexion; excessive use may cause narcotic condition
dandelion	leaf and root	when taken regularly adds a healthy bloom to the complexion and acts as a tonic to fortify the body systems; digestive, diuretic
elder	flowers	for asthma, chills, colds, fevers; induces sleep, promotes perspiration
fennel	seed	takes away hunger pangs, so is ideal for people on a diet; relieves flatulence
horsetail	stem	excellent strengthener of hair, fingernails and tooth enamel
juniper	berries	has a cleansing effect on the body systems, and is reputed to restore youthful vigour; builds up resistance; take for chest complaints, intestinal troubles, kidneys, nerves, diabetes; antiseptic, stimulant, diuretic. Warning: overuse can cause irritation and inflammation of the kidneys

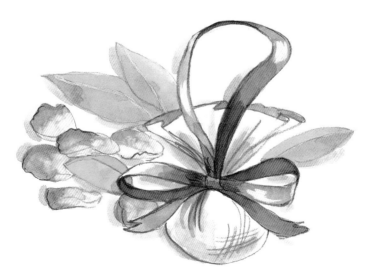

Herb	Parts Used	Application and Effect
kelp	whole plant	will help to take weight off the hip area. Take in combination with other herbs
lemon grass	leaf	helps to clear complexion and give skin a fine texture and healthy glow
lime (linden)	flowers	acts as a general tonic
lovage	seeds	use as a gargle for throat and mouth infections; aids digestion; stimulant
marigold (calendula)	flowers	for digestive problems; improves the complexion
marjoram marjoram and chamomile	leaf leaf and flower	for sore throats, colds; soothing promotes sound, soothing sleep; beneficial tonic for the system
marshmallow and malva	root and leaf	use as a treatment for teenage acne
nettle	leaf	contains vitamin D, iron, calcium and other trace elements. Use as blood tonic (purifier), to stimulate digestion; reputed to increase lactation in nursing mothers; for colds, sore throats (as a gargle); improves liver function; its astringent qualities are said to relieve urinary disorders and rheumatic problems

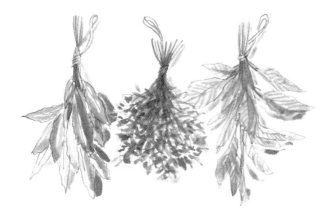

Herb	Parts Used	Application and Effect
oat straw	stem	aids in building strong fingernails, and eliminates split ends from hair
parsley	leaf	aids digestion; tonic, diuretic, relieves flatulence
peppermint	leaf	for colds, headaches, diarrhoea, flatulence, heartburn, nausea, indigestion, congestion, abdominal pain, cramps and vomiting; acts as a tonic; blend equal parts of peppermint, elder flower and yarrow for cold and 'flu
raspberry	leaf	traditionally recommended for expectant mothers for relief of morning sickness, to ease childbirth and assist lactation; said to tone up mucous membranes
rose	hip (dried)	for gall bladder and kidneys; source of vitamin C; diuretic
rosemary	leaf	tonic to freshen the breath; induces sleep, alleviates headache and strengthens the nerves
sage	leaf	cooled tea makes a soothing mouth rinse for inflamed gums and is a helpful gargle for sore throats; calms the nerves and acts as a blood tonic
silverweed	whole plant	cures swollen gums
sorrel	leaf	blood purifier
spearmint	leaf	prevents bad breath, is good for the gums, and helps whiten teeth
thyme	leaf	use the cool tea as a mouth rinse to freshen the breath; for coughs, colds, and sinus ailments; soothing
verbena (lemon)	leaf	refreshing and relaxing drink; ideal on hot summer days

Herb	Parts Used	Application and Effect
verbena (vervain)	leaf and root (dried)	mild sedative; soothing, digestive
violet	flowers	for headaches, insomnia, coughs, nerves; mixed with almond oil is a mild laxative; soothing
witch hazel	bark and leaf	use the cool tea as a gargle for sore throat, or a mouthwash for bleeding gums
wood betony	leaf	good general tonic; makes an excellent substitute for traditional tea — resembles the taste but is caffeine free

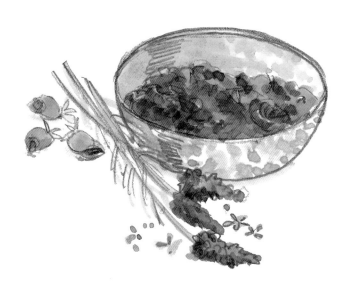

CHAPTER SEVEN
Fragrance

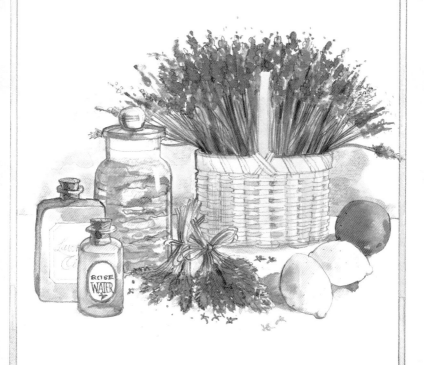

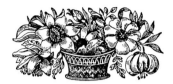

*B*ecause of its sophisticated technology, commercial perfume manufacturing is a science beyond the capabilities of the amateur. However, flowers and herbs can be made into delightful vinegars, colognes and perfumes. They will lift your spirits, make you feel special, and cool and refresh your skin. All that is required to make your own fragrances is basic kitchen equipment and easily obtainable ingredients. The techniques themselves are relatively simple and fun to experiment with.

Perfumes
❖

The range of perfumes you can create is really only limited by your imagination and the variety of scented plants you have available. The following examples should inspire you to experiment further and produce fragrances to suit your own tastes and preferences.

FLORIDA WATER
❖

2 cups fresh rose petals
2 cups (500 ml/16 fl oz) vodka
2 tablespoons whole cloves
2 tablespoons dried rosemary
2 tablespoons dried basil
2 cinnamon sticks
essential oils:
8 drops orange flower
8 drops lavender
8 drops rosemary
5 ml (⅙ fl oz) lemon

In a covered ceramic pot steep the rose petals in 1 cup (250 ml/8 fl oz) vodka for a week. In the other cup of vodka simmer the cloves, rosemary and basil in a covered enamel pot for 15 minutes, add crushed cinnamon, then leave to steep for 24 hours. Strain both cups of vodka and discard petals, herbs and spices. Mix solutions together and drip through filter paper 3 times; add remaining oils and stir well. Store in an airtight bottle.

EAU-DE-COLOGNE PERFUME

essential oils of:
3 ml bergamot
3 ml lemon
1½ ml orange flower
20 drops neroli
10 drops rosemary
200 ml (6½ fl oz) orrisroot perfume base alcohol (or vodka)

Mix all ingredients, drip through filter paper, and store in airtight bottle.

HUNGARY WATER

essential oils:
2½ ml rosemary
2½ ml lavender
750 ml (24 fl oz) vodka
250 ml (8 fl oz) orange flower water

Dissolve the essential oils in the vodka, mix with flower water, and store in an airtight bottle.

EAU-DE-ROSE

Unlike simple cosmetic rosewater (infused in water), this version is stronger and should be used sparingly, as it makes a potent perfume.

Two-thirds fill a wide-mouthed glass jar with vodka and add fresh rose petals until no more can be forced into the jar. Seal tightly. Allow the mixture to stand for 6 to 8 weeks, or until the aromatic essence has left the petals. Strain and store in an airtight bottle.

FLOWER PERFUME

Use any highly fragrant flower, such as rosebuds, lavender, jasmine or orange blossom, to make this old-fashioned perfume.

Place selected blossoms in a ceramic bowl and add just enough boiling water to cover them. Cover the bowl with a plate, steep until cool, and strain through muslin cloth.

Steep a cinnamon stick in vodka overnight, and mix equal amounts of the vodka and flower infusion. Drip through filter paper and store in an airtight bottle.

ROSE AND LAVENDER COLOGNE
❖

½ cup fresh scented rose petals
150 ml (5 fl oz) vodka
½ cup fresh lavender flowers
2 tablespoons thinly-pared lemon peel
2 tablespoons thinly-pared orange peel
150 ml (5 fl oz) boiling water

Steep the rose petals in the vodka in an airtight jar for 14 days. Put the lavender flowers, lemon peel and orange peel in a ceramic bowl and pour the boiling water over them. Cover and steep overnight, then strain through muslin cloth. Blend the infusion with the rose alcohol, drip through filter paper, and store in a tightly-sealed bottle. Leave for 7 days before using, shaking every day.

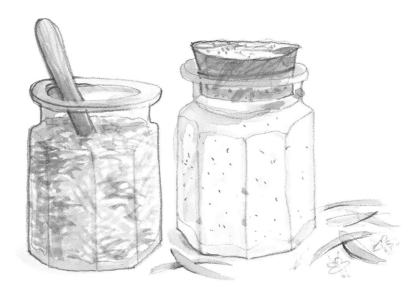

ROSE TOILET WATER

250 ml (8 fl oz) rosewater
20 ml (⅔ fl oz) orange flower water
750 ml (24 fl oz) vodka
essence of:
5 ml (⅙ fl oz) violet
1 ml jasmine
1 ml lemon verbena
essential oil:
5 ml (⅙ fl oz) rosemary
3 ml bergamot

Mix all ingredients thoroughly and allow to stand for a month. Drip through filter paper into glass bottles and seal tightly.

LAVENDER WATER

6 ml essential oil of lavender
30 drops essential oil of bergamot
570 ml (19 fl oz) vodka
140 ml (4½ fl oz) distilled water

Mix all ingredients and allow to stand for 10 days. Drip through filter paper and store in a tightly-sealed glass bottle.

Refreshing Skin Colognes

These are ideal for use on hot summer days and nights. They will give your spirits a lift by making you feel fresh and cool.

ELDER FLOWER SKIN FRESHENER

2 cups fresh elder flowers
500 ml (16 fl oz) boiling water
150 ml (5 fl oz) vodka

Put the elder flowers in a ceramic bowl and add the boiling water. Cover, steep overnight, strain through muslin and blend with vodka. Drip through filter paper and store in an airtight bottle.

LEMON COLOGNE
❖

During hot summers this cologne will not only refresh you, but impart a beautiful lemon scent.

9 ml essential oil of lemon grass
50 ml (1½ fl oz) essential oil of lemon peel
12 ml (½ fl oz) essential oil of orange peel
2 litres (64 fl oz) vodka

Mix together all the ingredients and allow the mixture to stand for a month. Drip through filter paper and store in a tightly-sealed bottle.

LEMON BALM COLOGNE
❖

4 cups (tightly-packed) fresh lemon balm leaves
2 litres (64 fl oz) vodka
1 litre (35 fl oz) distilled water
7 ml (¼ fl oz) essential oil of lime peel
15 ml (½ fl oz) essential oil of lemon peel

Steep the lemon balm in vodka for 14 days, and strain. Mix the lemon alcohol mixture with the distilled water and essential oils and allow to stand for 10 days. Drip through filter paper and store in tightly-sealed glass bottles.

VIOLET AND ROSE SKIN REFRESHER
❖

2 cups fresh violet petals
1 cup fresh rose petals
3 cups (750 ml/24 fl oz) distilled water
375 ml (12 fl oz) vodka

Prepare Floral Water (see Chapter Eight), then add distilled water after the process to make 750 ml (24 fl oz/3 cups). Mix thoroughly with the vodka, allow to stand for 7 days and then drip through filter paper into glass bottles and tightly seal.

Soothing Floral Vinegars

Floral vinegars are more astringent than floral scents made with alcohol. They are extremely refreshing when dabbed behind the ears and on the temples and forehead, and ideal to use after exposure to hot sun.

Vinegars will also soften facial and body skin, and can be used as a soothing compress to relieve headaches. Use neat or mixed with equal quantities of distilled water or floral water.

Flowers and Herbs to Use:
Basil, cloves, dill, scented geranium leaves, honeysuckle, jasmine, lavender, lemon verbena, rose, rosemary and violet.

1½ cups fresh flower petals or herbs
2 cups (500 ml/16 fl oz) cider vinegar or wine vinegar

Put the flower petals or herbs into a large, wide-mouthed jar. Gently warm the vinegar, pour into the jar, seal tightly and leave where it will receive plenty of sunlight for 2 weeks. Shake the contents every day. Strain the vinegar and store in tightly-sealed bottles. Dilute as required.

If the scent is not strong enough, repeat the procedure with a fresh batch of flowers or herbs.

SOOTHING LAVENDER VINEGAR
❖

125 ml (4 fl oz) lavender vinegar
250 ml (8 fl oz) rosewater

Mix the ingredients thoroughly and store in tightly-sealed bottles.

VINEGAR FACE WASH
❖

Apply directly to the face to ease that hot, sticky feeling on humid summer days.

40 ml (1½ fl oz) lavender or lemon verbena vinegar
250 ml (8 fl oz) rosewater

Mix thoroughly and store in a tightly-sealed bottle.

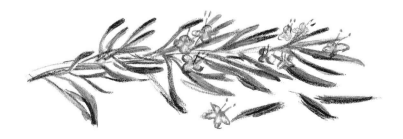

Lingering Fragrances

The following suggestions will help to make your natural fragrances last longer:

- Always apply to pulse points.
- Apply to several points, not just one.
- Don't skimp. Be generous and apply liberally so the initial lift of your fragrance is a little more intense than you actually want it to be.
- To avoid neutralising your fragrance, use unscented grooming products.
- Make your body powder and body lotion with the same scent as your fragrance.
- Scent applied to the inside of your wrists tends to be removed when washing your hands.

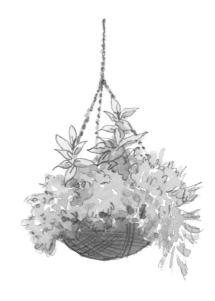

CHAPTER EIGHT
Extraction of Oils and Essences

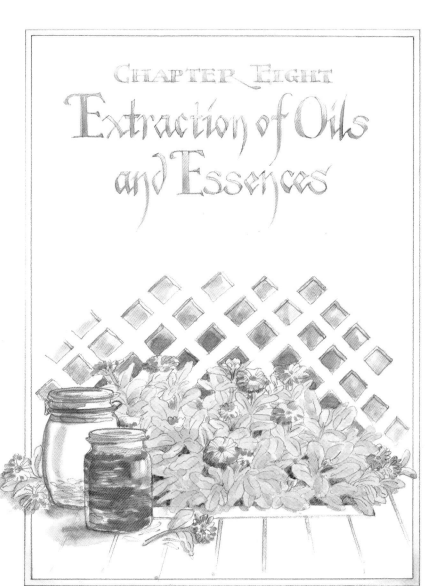

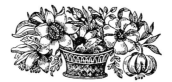

*V*olatile oils, the life force of all plants, contain the scent of the flowers, leaves, stems, roots or bark from which they come and have been used in cosmetic preparations for thousands of years. They can be used in beauty waters, perfumes, soap, creams, lotions, and added to your bath.

These valuable essences can be extracted in different ways: distillation and enfleurage (herbs and flowers) to give you a pure essential oil; by the use of a carrier oil; in alcohol or vinegar; by steeping or boiling the plant materials.

This chapter deals with different methods of extraction, all of which are easily carried out within the home.

Herb and Flower Oils

❖

Sun Distillation

This is based on the ancient method of extracting the precious attar (fragrant essential oil) of roses. However, all sweet-scented flowers, herbs and fruits will yield their aromatic oils by this process.

Place fresh flower petals or herbs in a large, wide-mouthed glass jar and cover with distilled water. (If using fruit, tear and bruise the skin first.) Seal the jar with plastic wrapfilm, ensuring that it is airtight, and leave it where it will receive hot sunlight every day.

When a thin film of oil appears, gently lift it off with cotton wool and squeeze it into a small glass bottle. Seal the bottle tightly, reseal the distilling jar and continue the process until no more oil appears.

CALENDULA (MARIGOLD) OIL
❖

Pure calendula oil can be extracted with just a glass jar and hot sunlight.

Tightly pack flower heads into a wide-mouthed jar that has a tight-fitting lid. Leave in the sun for several days until an oily orange fluid appears on the bottom of the jar. This is pure calendula oil. Repeat this process until you have sufficient oil.

Enfleurage

Choose fresh herbs or flower petals in the morning, after the dew has evaporated and they are at their most fragrant. Select only perfect specimens, discarding any damaged ones and keeping different types of herbs separated.

Place a layer of petals or herb leaves in the bottom of a small ceramic pot (such as a casserole) — never use glass or metal — and sprinkle a thin layer of coarse salt over them, repeating the procedure until the vessel is full.

Put the lid in place and seal tightly with plasticine or Blu-Tac. Leave undisturbed for a month in a cool, dark cupboard.

After a month, strain into a glass jar, squeezing all liquid from the mass. Seal the jar and leave it, where it will receive plenty of sunlight, for 6 weeks, so that any sediment will settle. You will now have a concentrated fragrant oil.

You can strain once more through filter paper.

BATH AND COSMETIC OILS
❖

These are not pure essential oils, as previously extracted, but merely fragrant oils, where the volatile properties of the plant have been extracted by means of an odourless vegetable oil. They can be used instead of fresh herbs in your bath or added to the various skin care preparations.

When being used to provide scent, add approximately twice as much as a pure essence; however, care should be taken and the oil added one drop at a time until the desired strength is obtained.

Use only highly aromatic flower petals and herbs, adopting the same gathering and selection procedure as for pure essential oils (see enfleurage above).

Spread the selected herbs or petals on a shallow tray and sprinkle a small quantity of non-iodised salt over them. Place a layer of the herbs and salt in a wide-mouthed jar and then a layer of cotton wool, combed out thinly and soaked in a suitable carrier oil, such as almond, olive or sunflower oil.

Repeat this procedure of alternating layers until the jar is full. Place the jar on top of a sheet of clear plastic and tie the plastic tightly over the top, enclosing the jar.

Leave in a sunny spot for at least 15 days, then squeeze the fragrant oil from the whole mass. Strain and store your fragrant oil in a tightly-sealed bottle.

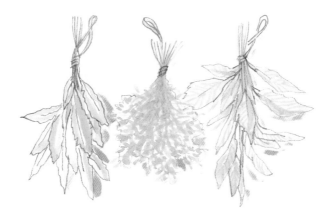

DRIED HERB METHOD
❖

Put two handfuls of dried flower petals or herbs in a large glass jar and cover with ½ litre (500 ml/16 fl oz) of carrier oil. Seal tightly, and leave in a sunny spot for 3 to 4 weeks, or longer if necessary. Shake the contents vigorously every second day.

Strain into a glass bottle and seal.

Keeping Herb and Flower Oils
Essential oils should always be stored in small, amber-coloured, airtight glass bottles, away from heat and light. Never keep mixed oils, and especially those made with a carrier oil base, any longer than two months because they begin to oxidise as soon as they are blended.

Herb and Flower Waters

The simplest herb water is made by steeping fresh or dried herbs in boiling water, and is known as a 'herbal infusion'. However, the bark and roots of a plant will not yield their properties by this process and must be extracted by a method called a 'decoction'. The delicate scent of flowers needs to be treated differently again, and can be obtained by a variety of processes.

Herbal Infusion
Place the selected herbs in a large ceramic bowl and pour boiling water over them. Cover and steep for 12 hours (overnight) for a strong infusion,

until cool for a weak infusion, or as otherwise directed, then strain through muslin and add required amount to recipe.

The following proportions should apply: fresh herbs 3 to 4 tablespoons, or dried herbs 1 to 2 teaspoons, to every 300 ml (10 fl oz) of boiling water

Herbal infusions can be made from one herb or a mixture of herbs, depending upon the requirements of a recipe or your particular needs.

Usually, most infusions will last only one or two days, unless kept in a glass bottle in the refrigerator, when they last up to a week.

To extend the keeping qualities of the infusions, add 5 to 10 ml/ ⅙ to ⅓ fl oz of vodka to every 300 to 500 ml/10 to 16 fl oz of infusion, or 3 to 4 drops of tincture of benzoin (friar's balsam) to every 300 ml/ 10 fl oz.

Decoction

Put the selected herbs in a stainless steel or enamel pan and add distilled water. Bring to the boil and then simmer for 30 minutes (unless otherwise directed). Remove from heat, cover the pan, and allow to steep for 10 minutes. Strain through muslin and add required amount to recipe.

The following proportions should apply: fresh herbs 3 to 4 tablespoons, or dried herbs 1 to 2 teaspoons, to every 300 ml/10 fl oz of distilled water.

Flower Waters

This will give you beautifully-scented water from any fragrant flower.

Put 4 tablespoons of fresh flower petals in an enamel or stainless steel pan and cover with 1½ cups (375 ml/12 fl oz) of distilled water. Bring to boiling point, cover and simmer for 30 minutes. Remove from heat, cool, strain through muslin, and squeeze any remaining liquid from the flower petals.

Repeat this process, depending on the strength and type of flowers used, up to four more times for greater potency. Add fresh flowers to the liquid and top up if necessary.

FLOWER WATER MADE IN THE OVEN

❖

Use 900 g (30 oz) of fresh flower petals or 600 g/20 oz of dried flowers. Put the flowers in a ceramic casserole, cover with distilled water, and place in an oven that has been preheated to 220°C/435°F. When the water reaches boiling point replace the casserole lid and leave in the oven for a further 15 minutes. Remove, allow to cool while covered, then strain through muslin.

Essential Oil and Water

A potent fragrant water can be made by adding 2 drops of pure essential herb or flower oil to 1 litre/32 fl oz of distilled water. Use to splash on your face and body or include in your bath water.

ROSEWATER PERFUME
❖

6 ml essential oil of rose
25 drops essential oil of bergamot
250 ml (8 fl oz) rosewater
750 ml (24 fl oz) vodka

Mix all ingredients and allow to stand in an airtight jar for 10 days. Drip through filter paper and store in tightly-sealed glass bottles.

LAVENDER AND ROSE TOILET WATER
❖

6 ml essential oil of lavender
140 ml (4½ fl oz) rosewater
570 ml (19 fl oz) vodka

Mix all ingredients and allow to stand for 10 days. Drip through filter paper and store in tightly-sealed glass bottles.

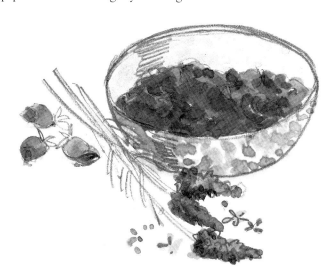

CHAPTER EIGHT ❖ 95

Keeping Herb and Flower Waters

All herb and flower waters prepared using the above methods can have their keeping qualities extended. Lavender, due to its natural antiseptic properties, has good keeping qualities, while other herbs will keep quite well if vodka or tincture of benzoin is added as directed under Herbal Infusion.

Should you make large quantities of fragrant water, the addition of alcohol will ensure that it lasts indefinitely. Add 1 part vodka to 2 parts fragrant water, stand for 12 hours, then drip through filter paper.

EAU DE COLOGNE TYPE PERFUME
❖❖

4 tablespoons fresh rose petals
1 cup (250 ml/8 fl oz) vodka
1 tablespoon fresh basil leaves
1 tablespoon fresh peppermint leaves
2 tablespoons grated orange peel
2 cups (500 ml/16 fl oz) boiling water

Soak the rose petals in vodka in an airtight jar for a week. On the seventh day crush the herb leaves, and steep, with the grated orange peel, in boiling water. When cool, strain both liquids, mix thoroughly together and drip through filter paper. Store in an airtight bottle.

Tinctures

Tinctures are made by steeping dried or crushed fresh plants in alcohol. All aromatic flowers and herbs can be used, and should be gathered in the morning when their fragrance is strongest.

Two-thirds fill a large, wide-mouthed glass jar with vodka. Add herbs or flowers until no more can be forced into the jar, and seal tightly. Allow the mixture to stand for 6 to 8 weeks, or until the aromatic essence has left the herbs. Strain, drip through filter paper, and store in a tightly-sealed glass bottle.

This type of fragrant preparation will last indefinitely. Add a few drops to your bath or blend one part tincture to two parts distilled water for a fragrant toilet water.

Herb and Flower Vinegars

❖

Vinegars have been used for centuries as bath additions and beauty tonics. They can also be used as the basis of a natural deodorant and facial toning lotion, and have a far more refreshing scent that floral waters made with alcohol, as well as softening both facial and body skin.

BASIC RECIPE

❖

1½ cups fresh flower petals or herbs
2 cups (500 ml/16 fl oz) cider vinegar or white wine vinegar

Put the flower petals or herbs into a large, wide-mouthed glass jar. Gently warm the vinegar, pour into the jar, seal tightly, and leave where it will receive plenty of hot sun for 2 weeks. Shake the contents every day. Strain the vinegar and store in tightly-capped bottles.

If the scent is not strong enough, repeat the process with a fresh batch of flowers or herbs.

Herbal vinegars will keep indefinitely, and can be added undiluted to bath water, or diluted and used as face wash, skin toner or deodorant.

CHAPTER NINE
Harvesting and Drying Herbs

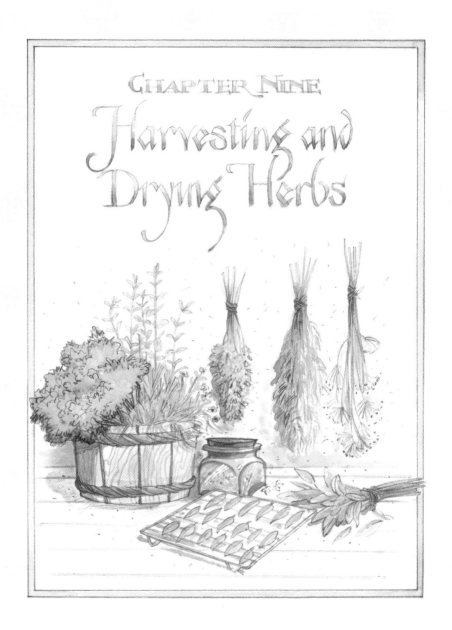

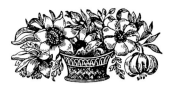

*T*here is nothing quite as tantalising to the nose as the fragrant aroma of fresh herbs. However, since many of them are annuals they are only available at certain times in the year. Therefore they should be preserved in a way most appropriate to their use.

A simple way to preserve herbs is to dry them, ensuring that they can be used all year round. So that they retain their colour and qualities, herbs have to be picked at the right moment and dried immediately afterwards.

By following these simple guidelines you will be assured of a ready supply of herbs throughout the year:

- gather herbs in the early morning when they are dry but before the sun has had a chance to draw out and disperse their volatile oils;
- do not pick herbs while they are still damp with dew or after rain;
- use a sharp knife, unless harvesting chives, which are best cut with a pair of good scissors;
- spread picked herbs out thinly on trays;
- do not collect more than you can immediately dry, as they will only deteriorate and lose their essential oil;
- avoid cross-flavouring by keeping different herbs separate;
- handle them as little as possible — herbs will bruise easily.

When gathering herbs it is important to know what and when to harvest.

Leaves — should be left attached to the stem and imperfect ones discarded. Volatile oils are at their peak just before the herb plant flowers, and leaves should be picked then.

Flowers — select only those which are unblemished and pick them when they are fully open.

Seeds — cut whole heads once they have turned brown and seeds are ready to fall. Leave on the stem.

Roots — horseradish may be harvested any time; all other herbs are gathered in autumn.

Because herbs contain about 80 per cent water, the object of drying after harvesting is to remove this water without delay to prevent the loss of their valuable and beneficial properties. They should be dried quickly with an even, low warmth — between 21°C/68°F and 32°C/90°F — and away from direct sunlight or wind.

What to Dry
The following table explains which herbs are best suited to drying and which parts.

Herb	Leaf	Flower	Seed	Root
angelica	x			
anise			x	
balm (lemon balm)	x			
basil (i)	x			
bay laurel	x			
bergamot	x	x		
caraway			x	
chamomile		x		
chicory				x
comfrey	x			x
coriander	x		x	
dandelion	x			x
dill	x		x	
elder (ii)		x		
geranium (*pelargonium*)	x			
juniper			berries	
lavender		x		
lovage	x			

Herb	Leaf	Flower	Seed	Root
marigold (*calendula*)		x		
marjoram	x			
mints	x			
nettle	x			
oregano	x			
parsley (iii)	x			
rosemary	x			
sage	x			
salad burnet	x			
savory	x			
soapwort	x			x
sunflower			x	
tarragon	x			
thyme	x			
verbena (lemon)	x			
vervain	x			
violet	x	x		

(i) Basil can be dried if laid out on a net in a warm, well-ventilated place. Otherwise use fresh at any time.

(ii) Elder — spread flowers out on a tray covered with net and keep in a warm, well-ventilated place until they feel papery to touch.

(iii) Parsley does not respond well to usual drying methods, but is successful when dried in a microwave oven.

Drying Herbs

❖

Air Drying

This requires no special arrangements: simply tie the herbs and flowers in bunches and hang them upside down in a dry, airy place, or spread them out thinly on net-covered trays and keep in a warm, well-ventilated place. Usually herbs will take 4 to 12 days to dry, sometimes longer.

Leaves — are dry when brittle, but will not shatter.

Flowers — are ready when petals feel dry and slightly crisp.

Seeds — after being removed from seedheads should be placed in the sun for a few hours.

Roots — should be dried right through with a soft centre.

Oven Drying

A less satisfactory method, since temperatures must be maintained below 32°C/90°F. Spread the herbs on trays and leave the oven door ajar to ensure ventilation.

Microwave Oven Drying

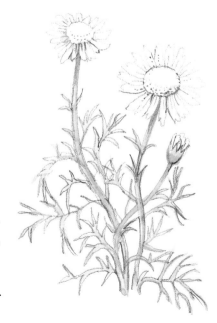

Most herbs, especially parsley, can be dried successfully in a microwave oven. It is advisable to do a few trial runs first to determine the best drying time. Turn the oven onto full power and place the washed herb on two layers of absorbent paper on top of an ovenproof tray. Usually it should not take longer than four minutes to dry each batch. Herbs with delicate, feathery leaves, such as fennel and dill weed, do not respond to this type of drying technique.

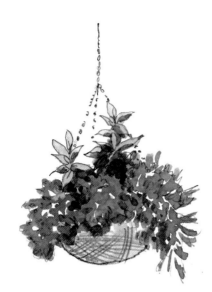

Screen Drying

This is a very simple process, requiring drying trays that are easy to make. They can be constructed from lengths of suitable timber, over which is stretched, and firmly secured, material such as cheesecloth or muslin cloth.

Spread the herbs one layer deep on screens, and leave them in a sunless, airy, warm room for about 10 to 14 days. For processing large batches, you may find it easier to use a dehydrator (drying cabinet).

Drying Cabinet

Herbs should be spread thinly on trays made from a wooden frame and covered with muslin cloth. These trays are then stacked in the cabinet with an 8 cm/3 in gap between trays for air circulation.

The drying space should smell only slightly of herbs. If there is too strong a smell you have too much heat. From time to time turn the herbs, and do not add any fresh ones until each batch is dry. Doing so will only add more humidity to the air.

Generally, herbs are ready once they are really brittle in leaf and stalk but still green in colour. To ensure even drying it may be advisable to swap the top and bottom trays during the process. However, be sure to do this without interruption.

The heat source for your drying cabinet can be a small fan heater or any suitable convection heater.

TIP: Construction of Cabinet:

The cabinet is no more than a simple wood-framed cupboard covered with three-ply.

Drying trays are made to fit the inside diameter, with wooden batten supports affixed to the inside of the cabinet to carry them. Reinforce your trays with a triangular gusset of plywood in each corner, and then cover with tightly-stretched muslin or cheesecloth.

To distribute the heat evenly a metal plate, about three-quarters the area of the bottom of the cabinet, is attached with heavy duty wire to the inside of the frame just below the bottom tray.

Storing the Herbs

When dry, herbs are rubbed gently by hand to discard the hard stalks — not too finely or they will lose their fragrance — and stored in clean, airtight glass containers. If storing them in metal bins, first place them in a linen or cotton bag. All containers should be kept in a cool, dark place so that the herbs retain their fragrance.

The following should be observed when storing herbs:

- thyme, sage and rosemary can be left on the stalk;
- seeds and flower heads should be placed immediately into airtight containers;
- roots should be ground like coffee beans and only stored in airtight glass containers.

If at any time the container shows signs of moisture on the inside, the herbs weren't dried sufficiently. Remove the herbs and place them on a sheet of plain paper and allow a further drying time. At the most, dried herbs will last only a year, so always remember to replace them the following season. An accurate way to check is to date your containers.

Grinding and Crushing Herbs

Some herbs are used ground, or crushed, as well as whole. Herb mixes are usually ground or crushed. Prepare large 'basic supply' containers of those you use most (in each state), and draw on these supplies to make up gift packages of single, or mixed, herbs at gift-giving time. This will also ensure that you have plenty of those herbs you need for your favourite recipes.

To crush herbs, tack a piece of cotton material over a wooden cutting board. Spread the herbs over the cotton and roll with a rolling pin. This will give you a coarse grind.

Herbs can be ground to a finer texture by rubbing them through a wire sieve. You can reduce them to a powder by processing in a blender or using a pestle and mortar.

Powdered herbs make ideal additions to cosmetic creams, especially those that have cleansing properties, or face packs.

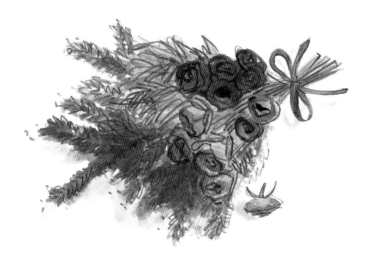

CHAPTER TEN
Herbs Forever

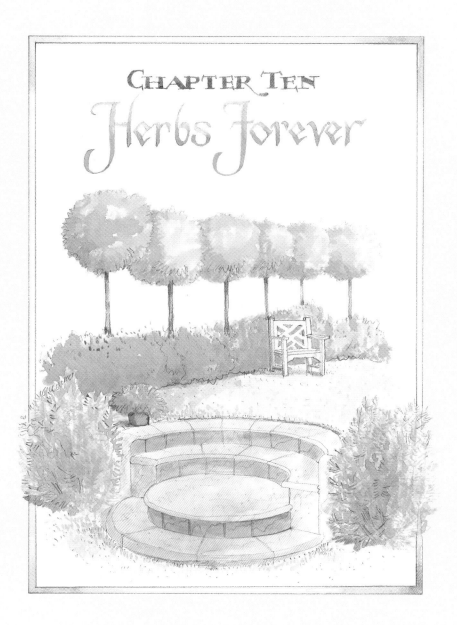

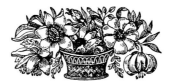

When it comes to creating a herb garden, size doesn't matter. It can be two or three hectares or a neat little pocket in the corner of the backyard. However, whatever the size, it must be planned, and the following factors taken into account:

- household requirements for herbs, either for cooking, craft, beauty products and medicines;
- your preference for herbs above other plants, or your desire to use them to create a garden, both practical and fragrant, with a truly individual character.

A few culinary herbs can be grown quite satisfactorily in pots, in an out-of-the-way corner, or incorporated into the vegetable patch. But if you are serious about herbs, and their fragrant cousins, they must be given their own garden area.

Unless you intend to grow commercially, herbs can be mixed with other plants to create an old-world cottage garden effect. This is both practical and delightful to the senses, with your herbs becoming the common thread throughout your entire garden.

The Cottage Garden

A potpourri of colour and scent that teases and tantalises the senses! A cottage garden involves the planting of perennials and herbs, intermingled with old world shrubs and fragrant plants, to provide a blend of colours and textures at all times of the year.

Created properly, an air of mystery will pervade, inviting the onlooker to explore each nook and cranny further. And it doesn't have to be large; being planted out correctly will give it an impression of distance.

Coarse-textured plants, such as the sweet-scented geraniums, and bright-coloured foliage will create the impression that they are close, while finely-textured plants, such as lavender, rosemary and various thymes, and dark-coloured foliage plants give the illusion that they are further away. So if you plant the coarse-textured, brightly-coloured herbs in the foreground, and the finely-textured, dark-coloured ones in the background, your garden will seem larger than it really is.

And of course a cottage garden should gracefully ramble around the house and yard, creating delightful pockets of both scent and colour, and a true old world feeling.

Appropriate Herbs and Flowers

In designing your fragrant garden, learning the growing habits and colour of the different herbs is important. You must know about the height of the plants you intend to grow, otherwise you might find that the tall herbs have been placed at the front of the bed, or near to, smothering the smaller and creeping herbs. Some herbs like sun, while others prefer shade; likewise with heavy and light soils. The more frequently-used culinary herbs can be grown close to the kitchen door, where they are handiest to the cook. These include parsley, basil, marjoram, thyme, chives, rosemary, dill and spearmint.

To enable you to plan your herb garden with greater ease, the following lists of plants are set out in fragrance, colour and height.

Old world Flowers:

Celandine	Columbine
Dames Violet	Dusty Miller
Daisies	Feverfew
Green Heliotrope	Winter Heliotrope
Hyssop	Heartsease
Larkspur	Leadwort
Motherwort	Night Scented Stock
Queen Anne's Lace	Southernwood
Spiked Speedwell	Marguerites

Perfumed Herbs and Flowers:

Azaleas	*fragrant varieties*
Basil (sweet)	*strongly aromatic leaves*
Boronia (Heaven Scent)	*wonderfully fragrant brown bells*
Cestrum nocturnum	*small shrub, evening scented flowers with a very powerful fragrance of almond-honey-musk*
Chamomile (lawn)	*fragrant ground cover*
Clary Sage	*aromatic leaves*
Dames Violet	*rich night perfume*

Daphne — *beautiful fragrance*
Dyer's Broom — *sweetly-scented flowers*
Evening Primrose — *soft fragrant night scent*
Fennel — *strong aniseed-scented leaves*
Frangipani (native) — *delightful fragrance*
Geraniums — *delightful fragrances of lime, peppermint, mint, rose and many others*
Golden Heliotrope — *fragrance of vanilla and custard*
Green Heliotrope — *vanilla ice cream shop fragrance*
Honeysuckle — *sweetly scented*
Jasmine — *richly perfumed*
Lavender (*L. spica*) — *very strong fragrance*
Lemon Balm — *smells wonderfully of fresh lemons*
Lime Balm — *distinctive, nose-twitching lime fragrance*
Lemon Verbena — *tangy, lemony fragrance*
Lime Blossom Bush — *vanilla scented*
Magnolia Port Wine — *heady, port wine-banana-fruit tingle fragrance*
Mock Orange — *stunning fragrance*
Night Scented Stock — *gentle fragrance at night*
Patchouli — *exotic, rich mint-sandalwood fragrance*
Pineapple Sage — *sweet pineapple-scented leaves*
Roses (all varieties) — *delightful perfume*
Rosemary — *fragrant evergreen*
Rue — *strong, highly aromatic herb*
Sweet Olive — *large shrub or hedge with a soft apricot-like fragrance*
Tarragon — *fragrant, shrubby perennial*
Tansy — *aromatic, dark green ferny leaves*
Tecoma (pink) — *blissful fragrance*
Thyme (ground cover) — *when trodden on releases a delightful fragrance to the air*
Violets — *highly-fragrant scent*
Wormwood — *delightful*

Colour in the Garden:

Blue Flowers

Ajugas   Alkanet
Borage   Columbine (some)
Comfrey   Daisies

Forget-me-nots
Lavender (some)
Leadwort
Savory (winter)
Violets

Hyssop
Larkspur
Rosemary
Spiked Speedwell

Lavender Flowers

Dames Violet
Savory (summer)

Geraniums

Lilac Flowers

Catnip (some)
Cat Thyme (some)
Larkspur
Snail Creeper
Violets

Catmint (some)
Golden Heliotrope
Mint
Vervain
Wood Betony

Pink Flowers

Clematis (montana)
Cone Flower (*Echinacea*)
Cumin
Frangipani (some)
Larkspur
Luculia rosea
Pink Hyssop
Snail Creeper
Tradescantia
Valerian

Comfrey
Coriander
Daisies
Geraniums (some)
Lavender (some)
Mint (some)
Pink Marjoram
Thyme
Tecoma (ideal for pergola)
Yarrow (some)

Purple/Mauve Flowers

Betony
Clary Sage

Chives
Comfrey

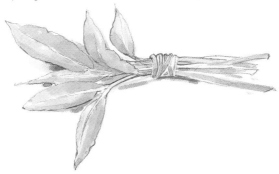

Green Heliotrope
Hyssop
Lemon Verbena
Mint (some)
Pennyroyal
Sage
Vervain
Winter Heliotrope

Heartsease
Lavender (some)
Lobelia (inflata)
Oregano
Pinks (pale mauve)
Thyme
Violets

Red Flowers

Bergamot
Geraniums
Lemon-Scented Myrtle
Pinks
Salad Burnet
Yarrow (some)

Field Poppy
Larkspur
Lobelia (inflata)
Red Valerian
Violets (some)

White Flowers

Anise
Caraway
Catnip (some)
Cat Thyme (some)
Comfrey (cream)
Creeping Tuberose
Feverfew
Geranium (rare)
Lavender (some)
Marjoram
Mock Orange
Oregano
Queen Anne's Lace
Sweet Cicely
Thyme
Violets
Winter Savory

Basil
Cardamom
Catmint (some)
Chamomile
Clethera (aboreta)
Daisies
Frangipani (some)
Hyssop
Lemon Balm
Mint
Old Man's Beard
Pinks
Rosemary
Tarragon
Tradescantia
Winter Heliotrope

Yellow Flowers

Agrimony
Daisies
Daphne
Dyer's Broom (golden)
Evening Primrose

Celandine
Dandelion
Dill
Elder (yellowish/cream)
Fennel

Frangipani (some)   Jack-of-the-Buttery
Lady's Mantle   Lime Blossom Bush
Lovage   Marigold (Calendula)
Rue   Tansy
Woolly Mullein

Foliage:

Grey
Catnip   Clary Sage
Costmary   Horehound
Lavender   Mugwort
Sage   Southernwood
Thyme   Wormwood

Variegated
Apple Mint   Comfrey (variegated)
Lemon Balm (golden)   Pelargonium
Thyme (silver and golden)   Sage (golden and tricolour)

Ground Cover Plants
Buttercup   Chamomile (*A. nobilis*)
Pennyroyal   Wormwood
Moneywort   Sweet Woodruff
Prostrate Rosemary   Thymes —
Golden Leaf Matting   Pink Flowering Matting
White Flowering Matting   Mauve Flowering Matting
Caraway Thyme   Shakespeare's Thyme
Woolly Thyme   *Thymus nitidus*

Hedge Plants
Catmint   English Box (*Buxus*)
Germander   Hyssop
Lavender   Rosemary
Sage   Santolina
Southernwood
Sweet Olive   Thyme
Wormwood

Climbing Plants
Akebia (*Trifoliata*)   Honeysuckle
Jasmines   Tecoma (pink)
Wisteria

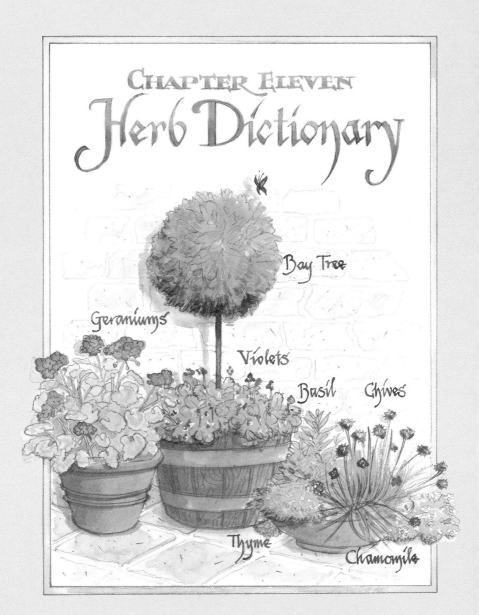

CHAPTER ELEVEN
Herb Dictionary

Bay Tree

Geraniums

Violets

Basil   Chives

Thyme

Chamomile

Agrimony *(Agrimonia eupatoria)*

A very pretty perennial, growing about 60 cm (2 ft) tall, with hairy, pinnate leaves and small, brilliant yellow, star-shaped flowers in spikes. Agrimony tea makes an excellent gargle for sore throats and is useful in the treatment of varicose veins. Its flowers will add colour to a fragrant garden and potpourri.

Alfalfa *(Medicago sativa)*

This plant is very rich in vitamins and minerals and can be used as an essential ingredient in mud packs for sensitive and delicate skin. It will not only cleanse facial skin, but also aid in the removal of dead skin, blackheads and grime from clogged pores.

Aloe Vera *(Aloe barbadensis)*

The juice of the aloe leaf has been used over the centuries in both medicinal and cosmetic preparations. It contains allantoin, proteins, minerals, vitamins A, B1, B2, C, E and K, and 18 amino acids, all of which give this herb unique properties. Included in cleansing masks and creams, its enzymes hasten removal of dead skin, and when added to moisturisers, it aids in the healing of damaged skin and stimulates growth in living cells.

Anise *(Pimpinella anisum)*

It is the small aromatic brown seeds of this plant, called aniseed, and containing the volatile oil, which are the most useful part. Chewing the seeds or drinking aniseed tea sweetens the breath and refreshes the palate.

Angelica *(Angelica archangelica)*

A tall, decorative herb with large, deeply-indented leaves and beautiful umbels of greenish-white or light green flowers. Taken as a tea it will act as a general tonic and soothe the nerves. When added to the bath it is both invigorating and rejuvenating, and acts as a tonic for the skin.

Basil *(Ocimum basilicum)*

Sweet basil is an annual growing about 80 (2 ft 8 in) cm tall, with light green, silky leaves and whorls of small, creamy white flowers. Taken as a tea it acts as a tonic that strengthens the body systems, and when added to a potpourri, its strongly aromatic leaves combine well with other herbs.

It's a delight to have in the garden; crush the leaves whenever you walk past it and the aroma will seem to linger forever. Include basil in perfumes, bath oils and vinegars.

Bay Tree *(Laurus nobilis)*

An evergreen tree with shiny, leathery, highly-aromatic, pointed leaves that are dark green on top and pale yellowish-green underneath. It is these aromatic leaves which make the plant important. Apart from its traditional use as a spicing agent, bay will combine well in a potpourri, add fragrance to a bath and comfort aching limbs, and in combination with chamomile, rosemary and rose, can be used as a facial steam that will cleanse and clear the skin.

Bergamot *(Monarda didyma)*

The colour, form and size of the bergamot flowers are amongst the showiest of all the herb blossoms. The plant is both decorative and fragrant, growing to a height of 60 to 90 cm(2 to 3 ft), with pom-pom type flowers ranging in colours from white, pink and mauve through to red.

Include it in the bath to revitalise the body and perfume the water; when dried it will add colour and perfume to a potpourri.

Blackberry *(Rubus fruticosus)*

Blackberry grows throughout Australia and can be found almost everywhere. It is rich in iron, vitamins and plant enzymes, and when taken as a tea will clear up minor skin disorders. The cold tea also makes an excellent gargle for sore throat swollen gums and loose teeth.

Borage *(Borago officinalis)*

This plant has a long history in herbal terms and has been cultivated for centuries. It is a sturdy, self-seeding annual, easily recognised by the fine bristly hairs that cover both the stem and large leaves and by its vivid sky-blue, star-shaped flowers. When used as a facial steam it improves dry, sensitive skin, and a cold tea compress applied to the veins of the legs aids in the prevention of varicose veins. Combined with chives or horsetail, and taken as a tea, it promotes the growth of healthy hair and strengthens nails.

Caraway *(Carum carvi)*

A biennial that grows to around 60 cm (2 ft) in height, with delicate, finely-cut and frond-like foliage and white umbrella-like flowers. It is the aromatic oil contained in the seeds of this plant that has the beneficial effect. And when taken as a tea or eaten it provides phosphorus, which is essential in maintaining healthy teeth and also aids in clearing the complexion.

Cat Plants
Catmint and Catnip — see Mints
Cat Thyme — see Thymes

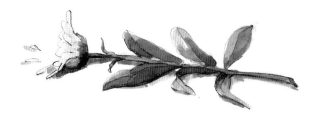

Cayenne *(Capsicum frutescens)*
A herb found in most homes throughout Australia, cayenne has been recognised for its beneficial effect on the entire digestive system and the circulatory system. Used in conjunction with other herbs it acts as a catalyst, accentuating their action by increasing their power and speeding up the beneficial effect.

Taken internally it is a natural source of magnesium and phosphorus, both of which are important elements in maintaining healthy teeth.

Chamomile — German *(Matricaria recutica)*
A low-growing, self-seeding annual with yellow and white daisy-like flowers that are used to make the popular tea. Included in the bath it has slight antiseptic qualities and is particularly beneficial to people with oily skin. Regular bathing helps to reduce and smooth out wrinkles, tone up relaxed muscles, and is very relaxing and soothing, thereby calming the nerves and promoting sound sleep. An infusion is ideal as a steam bath to cleanse and soothe the face, and is especially suitable for people with sensitive and delicate skin.

Taken as a tea, chamomile helps to soothe an overactive and tired brain. Added to herbal shampoos, or used as a hair rinse, it brightens fair hair and the oil makes an excellent scalp massage for unhealthy, lifeless hair.

Chamomile — 'Lawn' or 'Roman' *(Anthemis nobilis)*
An evergreen mat-forming perennial with fine bright green leaves and cheery daisy-like flowers. Lawn chamomile makes an ideal fragrant dense ground cover which is delightful to walk over barefooted.

Chervil *(Anthriscus cerefolium)*
Chervil is an annual which, in appearance, resembles parsley, and can be identified by its aromatic, pale green, fern-like leaves and small white flowers. Included in fragrant washing water it helps to smooth out wrinkles, and when taken as a tea, it is reputed to brighten dull eyes and clear the complexion.

Chickweed *(Stellaria media)*
Chickweed is a wild herb found growing all over the temperate world. It is a lush green, low-growing, self-seeding annual with tiny white star-like flowers. It can be used externally in a facial scrub for the treatment of acne or as a poultice over any skin eruption that needs to suppurate. A poultice is also an excellent medium for extracting any foreign matter from the eye without damaging the tissues, and is useful in conjunctival infections when grittiness and irritation are felt behind the eyelids.

Chicory *(Cichorium intybus)*
Chicory is a wild herb that grows in profusion in pastures and along roadside ditches and banks. When in flower it is a delight to the eye with its tall, cathedral-like spires of brilliant deep blue stretching toward the sky. A herbal tea made from the flowers is reputed to give the skin a healthy glow — but it should be taken in moderation.

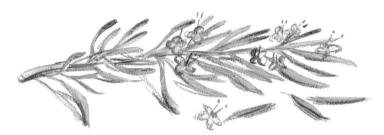

Chives *(Allium schoenoprasum)*

A bulb-forming perennial with thin, hollow, grass-like leaves. Chives are an excellent source of calcium and taken internally as a tea will help to strengthen nails and teeth.

Comfrey *(Symphytum officinale)*

A hardy perennial which dies back to the ground in winter, comfrey can be identified by its hairy, spinach-like leaves and stem and the bell-shaped flowers that grow in drooping clusters of blue, purple, pink or cream. Leaves should be picked in summer and, if required, roots dug up in autumn.

Comfrey is used in numerous herbal skin care preparations because of its unique healing properties. It contains vitamin B12, calcium and allantoin, and acts as a tonic for the skin as well as helping to smooth out wrinkles.

Coriander *(Coriandrum sativum)*

A hardy annual, of medium height, with umbels of pinky-white flowers and feathery, bright green leaves. A tea made from the seeds is excellent for purifying the blood, thus clearing the complexion. However, excessive use should be avoided as a narcotic condition may result.

Cotton, Lavender — see Lavender

Couchgrass *(Agropyron repens)*

A well-known and widespread grass in lawns throughout Australia. Taken as a tea, the roots of this plant are highly nutritive, extremely blood-purifying (which aids in clearing the complexion). Also strengthens nails and promotes glossy hair.

Dandelion *(Taraxacum officinale)*

This wild herb, found growing almost everywhere throughout Australia, is a virtual storehouse of vitamins, minerals, enzymes, proteins and other valuable elements, making it a wholesome plant food. Taken regularly as a tea it adds a healthy bloom to the complexion and acts as a general tonic to the body systems. And the root, dried, roasted and ground, makes an excellent caffeine-free substitute for coffee.

Dill *(Anethum graveolens)*

Dill is a decorative, fragrant member of the parsley family. It is an annual with delicate, feathery, blue-green leaves and has umbels of yellow, flat flowers. Included in herb vinegars it will soothe and soften facial and body skin.

Elder *(Sambucus nigra)*

An evergreen tree growing from 3 to 10 m (10 to 33 ft) in height, with rough, cork-like bark. It has delicate, dark green leaves with finely jagged edges and flat clusters of sweet-smelling, yellowish-cream flowers from which the dark red berries develop.

Elder water makes an excellent face lotion that is mildly astringent and particularly good to use after a cleanser. Made into a soothing ointment it will relieve facial soreness due to exposure to sea air. Included in the bath it is both healing and stimulating; in hand creams it will help to repair chapped skin and keep it supple; and when used in a facial steam it will tighten skin pores.

Eucalyptus *(Eucalyptus globulus)*

Eucalyptus oil is a good remedy for migraine headaches, and when added to the bath is delightfully aromatic and will help dilate capillaries for better circulation. When included in make-up remover it has a gently cleansing effect on facial skin.

Evening Primrose *(Oenothera lamarckiana)*

A tall, elegant plant, with large, yellow, papery flowers that grow on spikes up to 2 m (6½ ft) long. It is worth growing in the garden, and you will not go unrewarded when its soft fragrance is released to the air each evening at dusk. Made into an ointment, it will soothe rashes and skin irritations.

Fennel *(Foeniculum vulgare)*

A hardy perennial with beautiful, delicate, bright green feathery leaves and umbels of yellow flowers. It grows well everywhere, and is quite often seen growing wild along railway lines.

Fennel is valued for its ability to cleanse and smooth the skin and is included in many natural skin care preparations. Its gentle nature is excellent in cosmetics to be used on sensitive and delicate skin, and as a cold tea, it can be used to bathe sore and tired eyes.

Geranium *(Pelargonium denticulatum* — spicy; *P. fragrans* — nutmeg; *P. graveolens* — rose; *P. grosaroides* — coconut; *P. nervom* — lime; *P. odoratissimum* — juicy fruit; *P. torento* — ginger)

Imagine the exotic fragrances of nutmeg, spice, coconut, lemon, musk and mouth-watering lime! There is nothing more delightful than walking through your own garden after rain and being intoxicated by an assault of wondrous smells, or gathering any of the many-scented geranium leaves to perfume a hot bath. They can be included in herb sachets and pillows, or in potpourri mixes to add a touch of sweetness or spice, subtlety or headiness.

Geraniums vary in height and are shrubby plants with soft, hairy leaves that have deeply cut edges and loose umbels of varying shades of pink to lilac, red to lavender flowers.

There are many more varieties of sweet-scented geraniums than those listed: lemon, verbena, peppermint, apple, incense, pine, mint-rose, lemon-rose, and eucalyptus, to name a few. It is well worth spending the time and effort to search them out, as they make a wonderful fragrant addition to the herb garden.

Ginger *(Zingiber officinale)*

It is the root of this plant that has the greatest value. Add powdered ginger to your bath to open the pores of the skin and help rid your body of waste and toxins. As a tea it can sometimes be used as a hangover remedy because of its calming properties and ability to reduce nausea. People suffering from skin complaints are advised not to take large doses of this herb.

Honeysuckle *(Lonicera periclymenum)*

For centuries poets have sung the praises of the beauty and sweet perfume of honeysuckle: images that conjure up sunshine and lazy summer days. It is an old world plant that should be included in every herb garden, climbing beautifully up a dividing trellis or just rambling across the back fence.

Horsetail *(Equisetum arvense)*

A non-flowering, fern-like plant rich in silicate compounds as well as salts of magnesium and calcium, which help to correct absorption of the silica. Its high silica content can help skin complaints such as acne and eczema, and it is an excellent strengthener of hair, nails and tooth enamel.

Hyssop *(Hyssopus officinalis)*

An aromatic plant belonging to the mint family, which has been used as a medicinal herb for more than 2000 years. The flowers can be made into a tea that can be used to treat sore throats and catarrh, as well as skin irritations, burns, bruises, and insect bites. It makes a soothing wash for eye infections and the crushed leaves can be placed directly on to wounds to prevent infection and promote healing.

Jasmine *(Jasminum officinale)*

A strong, night-scented flower that releases its sweet aroma in the early evening. Although most people think of it as a climber, many varieties are weeping-arching graceful shrubs that also deserve a place in the garden.

The oil, when added to bath water, is reputed to be a relaxant, an antidepressant, and an aphrodisiac. It can also be used in an aromatherapy massage to treat respiratory problems and menstrual pain. The leaves can be made into a tea and used as an eyewash.

Juniper *(Juniperus communis)*

A small evergreen tree which, since ancient times, has been accredited with having mystical and magic properties. The ripe berries, when made into a tea, have a cleansing effect on the body systems, and are reputed to restore youthful vigour.

Juniper oil added to the bath, or used as an inhalation, is refreshing, stimulating and invigorating. It can also be used in an aromatherapy massage, therapeutic foot bath or aromatic shower.

Lady's Mantle *(Alchemilla vulgaris)*
A low-growing herb with greenish-yellow flowers found growing in clumps in damp, shady areas. It is easily grown from seed and when established will spread itself readily.

As a skin tonic it is effective against acne, and when used in a facial steam it has a cleansing and soothing effect on the skin.

Lavender — English *(Lavandula angustifolia; L. spica)*
Very similar in fragrance and form, these English lavenders are hardy perennial shrubs. Angustifolia has mid-blue to mauve flowers and L. spica has lovely true lilac flowers on graceful stems. Both will grow in full sun in temperate climates, but might need protection in warmer climates.

Dried flowers are used in potpourri and herb sachets, and the essential oil can be included in natural cosmetics, bath preparations and soap.

Lavender — French *(Lavandula dentata)*
A perennial shrub growing to around 1 m (3⅓ ft) high by 1 m (3⅓ ft) wide, which has narrow grey-green leaves with square-toothed edges. It is suitable for warmer climates and humid coastal areas and produces short, soft-stemmed, plump spikes of dark lavender flowers in the warmer months. It has a lavender scent (with just a hint of camphor) that does not have long lasting qualities when dried.

Lavender — Italian *(Lavandula stoechas)*
A hardy, dense compact shrub that is a very prolific flowerer, blooming in both spring and autumn. It produces spikes of dark purple flowers and is suitable for warm and humid coastal areas. Its uses are similar to those of English lavender, with a fragrance that is a blend of camphor and lavender with minty undertones.

Lavender Cotton — Santolina *(Santolina chamaecyparissus)*
A small woody shrub with silver-grey foliage and yellow button flowers that cover the plant in summer. It is hardy and drought resistant, preferring sun and good drainage, and makes an excellent garden hedge, growing to about 60cm (2 ft) tall. Dried flowers can be used in potpourris and moth-repellent sachets for wardrobes and drawers.

Lemon Balm *(Melissa officinalis)*
A lemon-scented herb that grows easily in the garden, smells wonderful, and can be used extensively in natural cosmetics, bath additives and herb pillows because of its soothing qualities. Balm tea aids the relief of migraine and when mixed with honey will soothe a sore throat. The fresh leaves are an effective mouth freshener, and also soothe insect bites and relieve toothache.

Lemon Grass *(Cymbopogon citratus)*
A semi-hardy, clump-forming grass that grows to about 1.8 m (6 ft) tall in warm

climates but less in cooler areas. Leaves can be used fresh or dry to make lemon grass tea, which helps to clear the complexion and give the skin a fine texture and a healthy glow. It is rich in vitamin A and the oil can be used in natural cosmetics to normalise the sebaceous glands, and to treat skin complaints.

Lemon Verbena *(Aloysia triphylla)*
This herb is a deciduous, frost-tender shrub that grows between 1 to 2 m (3⅓ to 6 ½ ft) tall. It has a wondrous, tangy, lemon fragrance, which is very refreshing when drunk as a hot or iced tea, or when a sprig is added to a glass of champagne. Dry leaves can be added to herb sachets and potpourris, or used to impart a delicious lemon scent in cosmetics and bath additives. It can also be used as an astringent tonic for oily skin.

Limeflowers — Linden Tree *(Tilia europaea)*
Cosmetically, limeflowers are used as an astringent to stimulate the skin and to help smooth out wrinkles. Made into a tea, they act as a general tonic and are a refreshing and nerve-soothing drink.

Linden trees need plenty of room to grow as they will reach heights of thirty metres or more, and live for more than a hundred years. In early spring the trees produce flowers with a strong smell of honey, which bees find very attractive. Dried flowers need to be treated with care, or they can quite easily lose the volatile oil they contain.

Lovage *(Levisticum officinale)*
Lovage is a herbaceous biennial with celery-like leaves, which prefers semi-shade. It will grow up to 1.5 m (5 ft) tall. An old-time aphrodisiac that seeds freely, lovage is often an essential ingredient in many stock cubes.

Cosmetically, it has a deodorant effect on the skin when added to the bath or applied under the arms. A cold tea is an excellent gargle for throat and mouth infections, or a soothing lotion for tired eyes.

Malva *(Malva rotundifolia)*
A common roadside weed that contains up to 17 per cent of essential minerals and has one of the highest vitamin A counts of any herb. Combined with marsh mallow it makes an excellent treatment for teenage acne, and can be taken as a tea or included in cosmetic preparations.

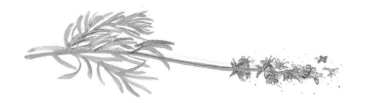

Marigold — Calendula *(Calendula officinalis)*
Calendula, also called English or pot marigold, is the one used in herbal preparations. It has flat-petalled, orange-coloured flowers, which are remarkably healing to the skin when applied directly or as an infusion.

It is excellent in the treatment of pimples, eases tired and aching feet, and is soothing and healing in a face mask for sensitive and delicate skin. Marigold oil, when rubbed into the feet, will relieve persistent soreness, and acts as an emollient in herbal cosmetic creams.

Marjoram — Wild Marjoram *(Origanum vulgare)*; **Sweet Marjoram**
(*O. majorana***)**
Wild marjoram, or oregano, is a small-leafed, creeping plant with purple flowers, and grows best in a warm, sunny position in well-drained fertile soil. Made into an infusion, it can be taken as a general tonic which will increase perspiration, and when combined with chamomile, it will promote sound, soothing sleep. Added to the bath it is a tonic to the skin and calming to the body. The essential oil can be used to relieve sore joints, arthritis, rheumatism and bruises, or placed directly on to an aching tooth.

Sweet Marjoram has similar properties, but since its flavour is not as strong it is more commonly used in cooking. It can be used as a tea to ease children's colic.

Marsh mallow *(Althaea officinalis)*
A decorative plant originally from marshy areas in China, but now growing wild in Australia as well as being cultivated. Taken as a tea, made from a decoction of the roots, it is a gargle for sore throats. It can also be applied to inflammations in the mouth and gums, and when diluted can be used as an eyewash. It can be combined with other herbs in lotions and creams to moisturise the skin, and is a suitable herb for the face, body and hair.

The leaves and root can be combined with malva to make an excellent healing cream for acne. Marsh mallow contains pectin, iron, albumin, asparagin, lecithin, enzymes, mallic acid and seven per cent of mineral ash, all of which treat and soothe both the physical and emotional trauma connected with acne.

Mint — Apple Mint *(Mentha suaveolens)*; **Curly** *(M. spicata 'Crispata')*;
Eau-de-cologne *(M. x piperita citrata)*; **Pennyroyal** *(M. pulegium)*;
Peppermint *(M. piperita)*; **Spearmint** *(M. spicata)*
All mints are perennial and well known for their aromatic leaves. They have white, lilac or purple flowers and will spread rapidly if not restricted. Some of the many varieties:

— apple mint is a very hardy plant in most soils, growing to about 40 cm (16 in) tall in spring and then dying back to the roots in winter. Leaves may be dried and used in potpourri mixes.

— curly mint is a rapid grower to 60 cm (2 ft), with hairy stems, wrinkled, broad, dull-green leaves and pale purple flowers. It is highly aromatic and the oil can be used as an antiseptic, while the leaves can be dried and added to a potpourri, or made into a refreshing tonic.

— eau-de-cologne mint has roundish, smooth leaves with a hint of bronze. Delightfully sweet, but its scent is better than its flavour. Its haunting aroma can be used as a basis for making a fragrant, natural perfume.

— pennyroyal is characterised by its whorls of pale purple flowers. It is a traditional lawn herb, which has a very strong scent that will repel insects, including fleas and ants, and can also be used in natural perfumes and to soothe bites and itching skin.

— peppermint has a slender, erect, deep red stem and longish leaves that are blushed with red and, on their underside, covered with fine hairs. Excellent as a repellent for insects or rodents, and when taken as a tea will help to relieve the symptoms of colds, 'flu and headaches. The oil can be applied directly for toothache or rubbed into rheumatic joints. Cosmetically, it can be used as an astringent to close facial pores, and when added to the bath it will soothe and ease itchy skin.

— spearmint grows to a medium height with long, narrow, pointed leaves and pinky-lilac flowers that appear in terminal clusters. Taken as a tea it prevents bad breath, is good for the gums, and helps whiten teeth. The cooled tea makes a refreshing mouth rinse, and a good skin lotion to improve the complexion and soothe roughened skin.

Catmints — Catmint *(N. faasenii);* Catnip *(Nepeta cataria)*
Catmint is a smaller-leafed, daintier plant, ideal for rockeries. It has a pretty wash of blue flowers and similar properties to catnip.
Catnip is a perennial shrub, traditionally thought to excite cats. It has attractive, aromatic, grey-green foliage and grows to around 60 cm (2 ft) tall. Taken as a tea it is both soothing and relaxing, and promotes a feeling of general wellbeing.

Mugwort *(Artemisia vulgaris)*
A common aromatic wild herb once used to flavour beer. As a bath additive it is helpful for tired, aching legs, and it also makes a good foot bath for tired feet. The fragrance of this plant will repel biting insects, and its fragrant oil (Amoise Oil) is used to give an exotic twist to expensive perfumes.

Nasturtium *(Tropaeolum majus)*
A creeping plant with bright red, orange and yellow flowers. Both flowers and leaves have a strong peppery taste, are high in vitamin C, and provide a valuable seasoning for people whose diet restricts their intake of pepper and salt.

Taken as a tea it is an antiseptic and tonic treatment for the blood and digestive organs, and helps clear the skin and eyes. A hot poultice made from the seeds can be used to treat boils and other skin eruptions.

As with many herbs, small amounts taken daily are far better than too much at once.

Nettle *(Urtica dioica)*
The stinging nettle is a hardy perennial found throughout the temperate regions of the world. It possesses many valuable nutritional and medicinal properties, such as vitamins, iron, protein, silicic acid, nitrogen, chlorophyll and other trace elements. It is of medium height and can be recognised by its dark green leaves covered with stinging hairs.

It is high in vitamins A and C, and made into a tea is a soothing gargle for sore throats. It can also be taken as tonic to purify the blood. Nettle is a useful ingredient in herbal products such as hair and skin tonics, and is particularly beneficial in controlling dandruff.

Oregano — see Marjoram (Wild)

Parsley *(Petroselinum crispum)*
One of the most popular and valuable of all herbs, parsley is rich in vitamins A, B, and C, and in iron and iodine.

Parsley is beneficial for the face, the eyes, the hair and as a deodorant. The cooled tea makes an excellent lotion for reducing puffiness around the eyes and for closing enlarged pores. Rubbed into the hair before shampooing, it makes the hair shiny.

Red Clover *(Trifolium pratense)*
The sweet-smelling, honey-tasting flower heads of red clover can be found growing in green paddocks everywhere from spring through to late summer.

When made into a tea they are soothing to the nerves and help to promote sleep, and an infusion can be used as a hair rinse or in the bath. Combined with dandelion and peppermint it makes an excellent substitute for China or Indian Tea.

Rose *(Rosa spp.)*
The species of rose most commonly used cosmetically are the old-fashioned Centifolia, Damascena and Gallica roses. However, the highly-perfumed, dark red modern varieties may be substituted.

Rosewater can be used on the face and the body and is cleansing, mildly astringent and hydrates the skin. Oil of rose can be used in face and body creams and lotions to impart a beautiful, delicate scent.

Included in the bath, rose petals will make the water fragrant and sweet, while also softening the skin. Dried, the flower petals and buds form the basis of most potpourri mixes.

Rosemary *(Rosmarinus officinalis)*
Rosemary is a well-known, aromatic, low-growing shrub, with spiky dark green leaves and clusters of small pale blue flowers. It is regarded as a symbol of remembrance, fidelity and friendship, and was believed to improve the memory.

Cosmetically it is cleansing, stimulating and restorative, and can be used as an infusion or as an essential oil. It is beneficial for the hair, as well as being a deodorant, a mouthwash and a bath herb. When put in bath water it will stimulate the circulation, soften the skin, relieve stiff joints and relax aching muscles.

Sage — Common Sage *(Salvia officinalis)*; Clary Sage *(S. sclarea)*

Sage has been used by the human race since ancient times for culinary, medicinal and cosmetic purposes. Ancient Egyptians revered it as both giver and saver of life, while Ancient Greeks thought it could render them immortal.

— common sage is a fast-spreading, medium-sized perennial shrub with hairy, grey-green, deeply-veined leaves and small mauve flowers. It can be used as a hair tonic and rinse, to help prevent hair going grey; a mouthwash for inflamed gums, sore throats and to keep teeth white; and as a tonic to close the pores of the skin.

— clary sage is a small, pleasantly-aromatic herb with very pretty flowers. In the Middle Ages its seeds were made into an eyewash, and today its highly fragrant oil is used as a fixative in perfumes. The leaves, when made into an infusion, can be added to the bath or used as an astringent lotion for oily skin.

Salad Burnet *(Sanguisorba minor)*

A small, hardy perennial with delicate lacy foliage and reddish flowers. For a constant supply of fresh young leaves, keep cutting the plants back, taking the first cutting when flower shoots appear. Use as a centrepiece in a low herb garden, or as a border plant.

Cosmetically, salad burnet can be used in skin-refining lotions, facial steams and acne preparations.

Silverweed *(Potentilla anserina)*

This wild herb belongs to the rose family and is worth seeking out. It has serrated leaves and yellow flowers like large buttercups.

Silverweed is a useful astringent, and when taken as a tea is helpful in treating skin disorders, swollen gums and loose teeth. The cooled tea can be used as a soothing, astringent lotion to close the pores of the skin.

Soapwort *(Saponaria officinalis)*

An attractive plant, soapwort is a hardy perennial of medium height with a

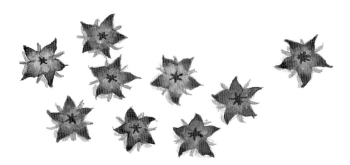

creeping rootstock. Its leaves are smooth and shiny and it blooms with large pink or white flowers. Leaves can be picked throughout the summer and roots dug in autumn and used fresh or dried.

The value of this herb is in its cleansing qualities. It can be included in natural shampoos or made into a bath washing liquid or shower gel to cleanse the body and wash itchy skin conditions such as dermatitis.

Sunflower *(Helianthus annus)*
The stout, erect sunflower is an annual which can grow to 1 m (3⅓ ft) or more in height. It has large, deeply veined, heart-shaped leaves that grow alternatively up its stem and bears one large yellow flower up to 30 cm (1 ft) across.

It is widely used for its oil, which is the richest and most beneficial of all the seed oils, and contains vitamins B, C, E and F. It is also rich in protein. The extracted oil is healing to the skin and can be used in natural cosmetic creams, or as a carrier oil for the extraction of essential flower or herb oils, as its aroma does not compete with those of the herbs.

Tansy *(Tanacetum vulgare)*
A hardy, clump-forming herb, dying back to the roots in winter to regrow in spring. It has attractive feathery leaves and clusters of bright yellow flowers, with a pungent scent of lemon and camphor.

Both the flowers and the leaves can be made into an infusion to externally treat pimples, sunburn, bruises and sore eyes.

Tarragon *(Artemisia dracunculus)*
French tarragon is a fragrant, shrubby perennial, growing larger each year, with widely-spaced, smooth, shiny leaves and clusters of whitish flowers. Pick leaves as required throughout summer and autumn, and cut mid-summer for drying.

Cosmetically it can be taken as a weak tea to cure insomnia and sweeten the breath, or dried and used in the making of potpourris.

Thyme *(Thymus spp.)*
There are many species of thyme, all descended from wild thyme. Its low growth and intense scent make it one of the herbs preferred for ground covers, as well as for flavouring and for use in dry perfumes and other natural cosmetic preparations. Thyme, in all its variations, is always worth growing, with its warm aromatic fragrance, attractive foliage and pretty flowers.

Thyme is also a powerful antiseptic, rich in thymol, and has many cosmetic benefits. It acts as an astringent and helps to clear spots and acne, cleanses, soothes and refreshes the skin, and when added to bath water as a strong infusion is excellent for skin diseases. As a scent herb, it is used in sachets, as a moth repellent, in rubbing vinegars, to make bath lotions, bags for herbal baths, to perfume soaps, and can be included in potpourris. The cooled tea makes an excellent mouthwash to freshen the breath, and when made into a tincture it can be used to cure fungal skin diseases such as athlete's foot. An infusion may occasionally be used as a facial tonic, as it encourages the flow of blood to the surface of the skin.

— Cat thyme (*Teucrium marum*) is an attractive plant with pungent, dainty grey leaves and masses of exquisite lilac, baby orchid flowers that bloom in summer. It looks very attractive growing in terracotta pots.

— wild thyme (*T. serpyllum*), or Mother-of-Thyme, is a low-growing ground cover with white, rose or crimson flowers.

— other varieties are:

lemon thyme (*T. citriodorus*)
golden edged lemon thyme (*T. citriodorus aureus*)
Westmoreland thyme (*T. serpyllum* 'Westmoreland')
caraway thyme (*T. herbaborona*)
pink flowering matting thyme (*T. villosus*)
white flowering matting thyme (*T. minimus*)

Violet *(Viola odorata)*

Sweet violet has roughly heart-shaped leaves and sweetly-perfumed deep purple flowers. Leaves and petals are both used cosmetically. They are soothing and cleansing to the skin, and gently astringent. Violet is suitable for all skin types, and may be used on the face and the body. The dried flowers can be used in potpourri mixtures, and will add a colour contrast as well as a hint of violet perfume.

Witch Hazel *(Hamamelis virginiana)*

Witch hazel is a small, deciduous shrub, well known as a skin freshener and for cooling the blood and allaying fevers. It is particularly beneficial for oily skin, and will reduce the size of large pores.

This herb is also useful as an underarm deodorant, to help smooth out wrinkles, to ease tired feet, as a compress for bruised and inflamed eyes, as a mouthwash for sore throats and gums, and as a douche for vaginitis.

Wood Betony *(Betonica officinalis)*

A wild herb, resembling a small aromatic stinging nettle, which has very nice dark green leaves and lilac-pink flowers. It is easily cultivated in the home herb garden and should be included.

Betony makes an excellent substitute for China and Indian tea, resembling the taste but being caffeine free. It also makes a good general tonic, is said to be effective against worms, helps to alleviate hayfever, and can be made into an ointment for use on sprains, cuts and sores.

Yarrow *(Achillea millefolium)*

Yarrow is a perennial which has a distinctive spicy scent, bottle-green feathery leaves and umbels of tiny white or pink flowers. It is an astringent and cleansing herb, and can be used in face masks, face scrubs, toners for large pores and oily skin, shampoos, and in a mouthwash. Combine with other herbs, otherwise it may cause photosensitivity.